"Daniel Dawes's groundbreaking and illuminating work on the political determinants of health will change how we think about the drivers of our health and well-being. It is one of the most important books in health policy to be written in years." —THOMAS A. LaVEIST, PhD, Tulane University School of Public Health and Tropical Medicine

"Daniel Dawes makes an engaging and important contribution to the health equity discourse with this book. He is also one of the few people in the country who could make this contribution. Because Dawes has been intimately engaged in the workings of government, he has a deep firsthand understanding of the political determinants of health. Moreover, he has a sweeping view of the historical movements that have contributed to the complexities of the American health care system. Dawes brings all of these threads to bear in this book and manages to make them relevant to the health equity movement today." —DAYNA BOWEN MATTHEW, JD, PhD, University of Virginia Law School

"Daniel Dawes insightfully argues that we have to be mindful of more than the social determinants of health. More specifically, he indicates that the political determinants of health are actually far more impactful and can be far more insidious when not properly addressed, given that the American political process is the foremost avenue for implementing change. He demonstrates that many challenges recognized as social determinants are the result of political determinants. I commend Professor Dawes for not only creating a detailed framework that outlines the political determinants of health but also providing us with timely enlightenment about the challenges that we are facing." —DAVID R. WILLIAMS, PhD, MPH, Harvard T.H. Chan School of Public Health

"Daniel Dawes presents another thought-provoking book showing us why addressing social determinants of health, while critically important, is merely nibbling around the edges of the problem. This book lays the groundwork for a transformation in how we think about advancing health equity by tackling the political determinants of health." —BRIAN SMEDLEY, PhD, American Psychological Association

"I have used Daniel Dawes's prior work, *150 Years of ObamaCare*, in my classes for the past three years. The book provided the students with a solid foundation and important insight into the history of the Affordable

Care Act and the US health equity movement. Dawes has now followed that with another groundbreaking book. In *The Political Determinants of Health*, he unveils a trailblazing model built on the latest evidence, clearly identifying the factors vital to any effective effort to address health inequities. The political determinants of health are key to understanding the myriad factors that contribute to inequities faced by underserved and marginalized communities. And they highlight a basic reality—that public health is inherently political. Dawes presents a road map for addressing the factors at the root of health outcomes in this country. This engaging book is a must-read for community members; policy makers; health professionals; social services professionals; behavioral health, public health, and health care leaders; advocates; academics; and future health professionals." —MARTHA MOORE-MONROY, MA, Mel and Enid Zuckerman College of Public Health, University of Arizona

"Politics shapes policy and policy impacts health. This text takes an insightful look at politics as a societal factor that determines public health. It is an essential read for anyone who strives to make the United States among the healthiest nations." —GEORGES C. BENJAMIN, MD, American Public Health Association

"The social determinants of health were an important advancement in our understanding of health. Now Daniel E. Dawes takes our understanding even further by developing a multidisciplinary framework explaining how policy and politics are tremendous drivers of the social conditions that affect all communities in a positive and negative way. Indeed, to truly address health, mental health, and substance use inequities, we need to understand their origins and their impact on the equitable distribution of opportunities and resources. *The Political Determinants of Health* does just that!" —OCTAVIO N. MARTINEZ Jr., MD, MPH, Hogg Foundation for Mental Health, The University of Texas at Austin

"This book shines a light on one of the most important aspects of modern life that impacts our nation's health. The role of politics and how it can diminish or worsen health equity has not been fully articulated in such a cohesive manner. This book will not only become an important guide for understanding health equity in America but will also serve as an essential tool for academic training and mentoring in higher education." —MARIO HERNANDEZ, PhD, University of South Florida

"Daniel E. Dawes elucidates a critical front in the drive to advance health equity: political determinants of health. Wise public policies and public support are essential to dismantle the structural drivers of inequities and create payment reforms that support and incentivize the tailored care that reduces health disparities." —MARSHALL H. CHIN, MD, MPH, University of Chicago Pritzker School of Medicine

"According to the World Health Organization, the distribution of money, power, and resources at the global, national, and local levels is what ultimately shapes our health and survival. This puts health, health care, and health equity squarely in the political domain. By shining a powerful light on the political determinants of health, Dawes compels us to face critical drivers of health and well-being in the United States today." —LAUDAN ARON, MA, Urban Institute

"Daniel E. Dawes continues to disrupt dominant narratives in this timely, groundbreaking book. So much of what creates and determines health happens outside of the doctor's office and hospital walls. Dawes pushes us all to move beyond our comfort zone of solely elevating the social and structural determinants of health and helps us to better understand the political drivers that produce optimal health for some and inequities for others." —ALETHA MAYBANK, MD, MPH, Chief Health Equity Officer and Vice President, American Medical Association

"Daniel Dawes forces a conversation that we can no longer afford to ignore with this impressively original and powerful book. In *The Political Determinants of Health*, readers will be challenged, motivated, and inspired to adopt a more expansive view of the role that political determinants play on our nation's health. Arguably the most important book written on the driving force that has prevented us from realizing health equity in America and around the world." —PATRICK J. KENNEDY, former congressman, founder of The Kennedy Forum, author of *A Common Struggle: A Personal Journey through the Past and Future of Mental Illness and Addiction*

"I was immediately struck by Daniel Dawes's insights in *The Political Determinants of Health*. This new concept will deepen the space loosely captured by structural determinants of health with a more foundational anchor." —MARGARET P. MOSS, JD (Hidatsa/Dakota), Director, First Nations House of Learning; School of Nursing, University of British Columbia

"In his latest book, Daniel Dawes, a leader on health inequalities in the United States, takes a critical look at the work on the margins of the 'social determinants of health.' He pushes back, arguing that political determinants of health are the fundamental issue, requiring a global answer to begin to achieve health equity. I'm looking forward to sharing this book with my students." —CAROLYN A. POINTER, JD, Southern Illinois University School of Medicine

"Daniel Dawes takes us further upstream to examine one of the most influential drivers that shape the health profile of our nation. *The Political Determinants of Health* offers invaluable insights for addressing the political, social, and economic factors that continue to adversely impact the health of diverse populations." —JANICE PHILLIPS, PhD, RN, CENP, FAAN, Director of Nursing Research and Health Equity, Rush University Medical Center, associate professor, Rush University College of Nursing

"In this riveting book, Dawes shifts behavioral health to the forefront and elucidates the limitations of our current approaches to addressing the determinants of health and how such approaches fall short in resolving the structural inequalities deep within our society." —ARTHUR C. EVANS, PhD, former Commissioner, Philadelphia Department of Behavioral Health and Intellectual disAbility Services

"*The Political Determinants of Health* provides a powerful lens through which to examine the structures, processes, and outcomes that account for unfair variations in health conditions among different groups. Because the United States is one of the most influential actors on the global stage, the insights from this in-depth study will illuminate our understanding of the pervasive inequities affecting health systems around the world. This is a must-read for everyone who wants to be a transformative force for global health equity." —JULIO FRENK, MD, PhD, President and professor of Public Health Sciences, University of Miami

The Political Determinants of Health

The Political Determinants of Health

Daniel E. Dawes

Foreword by David R. Williams

Johns Hopkins University Press / Baltimore

© 2020 Johns Hopkins University Press
All rights reserved. Published 2020
Printed in the United States of America on acid-free paper
9 8 7 6 5 4 3 2 1

Johns Hopkins University Press
2715 North Charles Street
Baltimore, Maryland 21218-4363
www.press.jhu.edu

Library of Congress Cataloging-in-Publication Data

Names: Dawes, Daniel E., 1980- author. | Williams, David R. (David Rudyard),
    1954- writer of foreword.
Title: The political determinants of health / Daniel E. Dawes ; foreword by
    David R. Williams.
Description: Baltimore : Johns Hopkins University Press, [2020] | Includes
    bibliographical references and index.
Identifiers: LCCN 2019033942 | ISBN 9781421437897 (paperback) |
    ISBN 9781421437903 (ebook)
Subjects: MESH: Social Determinants of Health | Politics | Healthcare Disparities |
    Health Equity | Legislation, Medical—history | United States
Classification: LCC RA425 | NLM WA 30 | DDC 362.1—dc23
LC record available at https://lccn.loc.gov/2019033942

A catalog record for this book is available from the British Library.

*Special discounts are available for bulk purchases of this book. For more information,
please contact Special Sales at specialsales@press.jhu.edu.*

Johns Hopkins University Press uses environmentally friendly book materials,
including recycled text paper that is composed of at least 30 percent post-consumer
waste, whenever possible.

To all who strive for a more healthy, equitable, and inclusive society

Contents

Foreword

Conflating the social determinants of health and the social processes that shape these determinants' unequal distribution can seriously mislead policy. . . . Policy objectives are defined quite differently, depending on whether the aim is to address determinants of health or determinants of health inequities.
—*O. Solar and A. Irwin,* A Conceptual Framework for Action on the Social Determinants of Health

In every great movement or struggle, the momentum of the cause eventually reaches a critical inflection point. At this point, stakeholders have to confront the reality that their efforts and strategies will effectively carry them toward achieving their goal or that circumstances require a new strategy to move forward. Today, America again finds itself at a moment of reckoning in its fight for health equity. Both America's history and its social and political forces have created a momentum propelling us and the global community toward this point. Yet, the fight is far from over. As we survey today's landscape, we can see that many hard-fought historical battles have netted gains, but we can also see setbacks that have challenged generations of health equity champions. For the health equity movement to capitalize on this contemporary moment, we have to recognize, address, and effectively combat the critical forces operating to the detriment of health and health equity. This book focuses on the structural inequities plaguing our society, while endorsing a new model for identifying their sources and strategically addressing them.

America is the undisputed world leader in many areas of evaluation, and most other countries look to us as exemplary on many different issues. However, we are not the healthiest people, even though we certainly should be, given our yearly per capita expenditure on health care—more, per person and absolutely, than in any other developed country.

According to the World Bank, half the annual expenditures worldwide on medical care are spent in the United States. We represent fewer than 5 percent of the world's population, consume one half of its medical resources, yet we still rank near the bottom of industrialized countries for health. Why are we receiving such a poor rate of return? More importantly, why are we comfortable with these outcomes? Published research has exhaustively answered the first question. More tellingly, an answer to the second question can be found in academic journals. But, by reframing the context of the problem, Daniel Dawes has succinctly answered both questions: one needs to look no further than the political determinants of health.

It is increasingly recognized that the social determinants of health are the most fundamental drivers of population health and health equity. While understanding what the social determinants of health entail is vital, we must also be willing to address these determinants (the causes of the causes). We have to advocate for, and implement effective strategies to address, the social determinants of health on the personal, clinical, community, and systemic levels. To achieve lasting change, we have to understand and confront the multiple intersecting factors at play. However, Dawes insightfully argues that we have to be mindful of more than the social determinants of health. More specifically, he indicates that the political determinants of health are actually far more influential and can be far more insidious when they are not properly addressed, given that the American political process is the foremost avenue for implementing change. He demonstrates that many challenges recognized as social determinants are in fact the result of political determinants. These political determinants are often masked as social determinants because it is more palatable to do so. I commend Dawes for not only creating a detailed framework that outlines the political determinants of health but also providing us with timely enlightenment about the challenges we are facing. Once we clearly understand what the political determinants are and how they intersect with health policy, we will be much more prepared to effectively harness the political process to implement needed changes.

America has a long history of tireless advocacy to create greater equity in society and in health. In recent years, we have seen signs of progress, such as the implementation of the Affordable Care Act, but we are also witnessing significant setbacks and inertia. There is increasing recognition of the need to address historical disparities, and phrases such as "social determinants of health," "health disparities," and "health equity" are losing their stigma. At the same time, evidence of persisting and sometimes widening disparities continues to accumulate. We cannot allow the rhetoric of addressing disparities to tempt us to rest on our laurels. Now is the time to address unfinished business with renewed vigor and to keep pressing forward toward further transformation of the health equity movement.

Senator Robert F. Kennedy once said, "Each time a man stands up for an ideal, or acts to improve the lot of others, or strikes out against injustice, he sends forth a tiny ripple of hope, and crossing each other from a million different centers of energy and daring those ripples build a current that can sweep down the mightiest walls of oppression and resistance."[1] Mighty walls of oppression and resistance face us as Americans. The political determinants of health and their impact on achieving health equity have erected some of the more powerful, yet rarely recognized and discussed walls of resistance. The lessons in this book send out clear ripples of hope that can create new tools and momentum to improve health outcomes of untold millions of Americans and to reduce and ultimately eliminate inequities in health.

The health equity movement is just that: a movement of people committed to advancing health equity for all communities. It requires the participation and unwavering commitment of all of us, working together to address all the determinants of health and advocating for improving the quality of life for those who have been historically ignored and excluded from opportunities afforded other privileged groups. With leaders like Daniel Dawes and his innovative approach to addressing structural inequities, I believe that the mighty walls of oppression and resistance that we currently face can be overcome and that the fight for health equity can serve as a desperately needed critical inflection point to provide justice for all and elevate America to its rightful place among the world's leaders.

David R. Williams
Florence Sprague Norman and Laura Smart Norman Professor of
Public Health
Chair of the Department of Social and Behavioral Sciences
Harvard T.H. Chan School of Public Health

Professor of African and African American Studies and Sociology
Harvard University

The Political Determinants of Health

1

The Allegory of the Orchard
The Political Determinants of Health Inequities

The care of human life and happiness, and not their destruction, is the first and only legitimate object of good government.—*"Thomas Jefferson to the Republicans of Washington County, Maryland, 31 March 1809"*

The movement to bolster health equity has heavily focused on health disparities, which are differences in health outcomes among population groups. However, not as much attention has been given to understanding the factors, systems, or structures (laws and policies) that create, perpetuate, or exacerbate these differences, many of which are unfair, avoidable, and remediable. Today, researchers recognize that there are multiple, interacting, complex determinants of health, including social, behavioral, environmental, and economic factors, which collectively affect your overall health and your ability to achieve health equity.

More attention has been spent on the social and economic forces affecting health equity,[1] the notion of extending to all people a fair opportunity to attain their optimal level of health and eliminating barriers that disadvantage people from achieving this opportunity. Girding all of the health determinants is one that rarely gets addressed but which has power over all aspects of health: the political determinants of health. Before becoming immersed in the complexities of the political determinants of health and the vast and systemic nature of intractable health inequities that have plagued our society, let me tell you a story that conveys the history of political actions and inactions that have resulted in health inequities in the United States of America.

The Farmer
A farmer sought to acquire new land in hopes of establishing an orchard and thus increasing his wealth. On his journey, he came upon a

plot that, though not perfect, he found suitable for his needs. One portion of the land was a bit rocky, another part of the land had poor soil, while a third part of the land had nutrient-rich soil. Despite its flaws, he felt he could work with this land and establish a thriving orchard.

As he surveyed the landscape, he found a beautiful tree that he had never seen before. The tree was well established in the nutrient-rich soil as evidenced by its size. Its limbs magnificently twisted and turned reaching across the landscape. The tree was not only majestic but also bore delicious fruit and sheltered the local wildlife. However, the farmer did not see any advantage in allowing the tree to take up valuable space on his new plot of land. So, he and his workers gathered all the fruit and dug up the tree, moving it to a corner of the land where it would be out of his way and eventually forgotten.

The Beginning

With the massive tree out of sight and six seeds in his pocket, the farmer was ready to cultivate his orchard. In the cool fall air, he planted two of the seeds in the rich soil where the tree once stood. He took his time digging the holes for the seeds, measuring the depth of the holes, and carefully placing the seeds. He thoughtfully added fertilizer and watered the seeds—after all, these seeds were on prime land, and he reasoned they deserved his full attention because they would likely yield his best crop.

After taking much time to establish the first two seeds, he commenced planting the next two seeds in the far less fertile soil. He dug holes for the seeds but did not feel the need to measure the depth as he had done earlier. He then used what little remaining fertilizer he had left after planting the first two seeds, and quickly watered the second set of seeds, as it was now beginning to get dark and he needed to plant the remaining seeds. Realizing that he had little time before the sun would set, he rushed to plant the final two seeds in the rocky soil, where he neglected to add the fertilizer or water them. Night fell and the farmer ended his day, eagerly anticipating what the spring would bring when the seeds would begin to germinate after the cold weather.

When spring arrived, the farmer readied his workers. Soon, they began to see the seedlings emerge, but the results were not what the farmer had hoped for. Of the two seeds that were planted in the rocky area, one never germinated a plant, but the other one somehow grew despite its circumstances. This seedling was weak and feeble, but it seemed determined to survive. The two seeds in the poor soil both germinated, but one soon shriveled up after breaking the soil, and the other continued growing, managing somehow to pull what little nutrients it could from the depleted soil. The two seeds in the rich soil broke through the soil and began flourishing quickly, producing fresh, tender, and bright green leaves, reaching up to the sun's warmth. Of the six original seeds, only four survived and matured into small trees: two in the nutrient-rich soil, one in the poor soil, and one in the rocky soil.

The Middle

The trees continued to grow through the spring and summer as the farmer patiently waited to someday reap his harvest. One warm evening, as the summer came to a close, a raging storm appeared out of nowhere and tore into the orchard. When the farmer went out to check on his orchard, he found that one of his four remaining trees had been struck by lightning, splitting it in two, leaving a limp and lifeless tree in the rocky soil.

The farmer now had only three remaining trees: two in the nutrient-rich soil and one in the nutrient-poor soil. Every few months, the farmer and his workers sprayed the trees with pesticide to prevent bugs from consuming the leaves. Nevertheless, the tree in the poor soil struggled. Some days the tree appeared vibrant and healthy, and the workers were sure the tree would produce great fruit. Other days the tree's young limbs drooped, seeming almost unable to bear the weight of its own leaves. The farmer noticed that this tree was struggling and instructed his workers to fertilize the ground. In obedience, the workers added the fertilizer, hoping it would keep the tree strong as the winter approached. When the cold weather set in, it was clear that the fertilizer was helping to keep the tree alive, but they were unsure what would happen when spring arrived. The farmer was expecting these trees to produce their first crop.

After a long winter, spring finally arrived and the farmer set out to examine his orchard. The two trees in the nutrient-rich soil were strong, their branches thick and sturdy, their fresh leaves glistening with morning dew. They were healthy, and the fruit they bore was large and sweet. The farmer was pleased. He had invested a great deal into these trees, and it was paying off. The farmer only had one more tree left to examine, the tree in the poor soil that had struggled the previous year. The tree was small, its limbs were weak, but, nevertheless, the tree was resilient. The fruit on the tree was small, and the farmer believed that this tree was not going to produce as much as his other two trees. In June, in a final attempt to redeem the tree, the workers irrigated the soil around it, hoping to avoid a low yield in the months to come. However, by late summer, the farmer did not see the results he had hoped for, despite his half-hearted and late attempts, and he decided not to invest anymore effort into helping this tree achieve its potential.

The farmer did not realize that the source of the tree's problem was underground where bugs had begun to gnaw at the roots. Instead of conducting a thorough examination of this tree to figure out the source of its problem or providing what it needed, when it needed it, and in the amount it needed, the farmer determined it was not worth the extra investment to help this tree realize its optimal level of health. Had he thoroughly examined the tree, he would have been able to address the needs of the tree and reap the benefits. The farmer, however, was hasty and otherwise preoccupied with the trees in the nutrient-rich soil.

Fortunately for the farmer, he received a letter from a dear friend, an arborist who specialized in studying and caring for trees. His friend wrote inquiring whether he could visit the farmer's orchard. The farmer quickly responded: his old friend was free to visit his farm and look at his trees. On receiving the farmer's reply, the arborist arranged to visit the new orchard, planning to arrive at the farm before winter. When he reached the farm, he was shocked that the farmer had so few trees. The farmer left his friend to examine his trees.

The arborist first examined the two healthy trees in the rich soil, finding them to be healthy and strong. He then examined the struggling tree in the poor soil. He was amazed that, despite the subpar conditions, the tree had managed to stay alive and even produce fruit. He recognized that this tree was indeed strong but that it had been weakened by neglect. Recognizing the inherent strength in the tree he realized that it would be a perfect specimen to study. The tree was obviously not the farmer's priority and was already producing so much less because of the harsh conditions that he felt it was best to use the tree to glean valuable information to benefit the other trees. He began experimenting with the struggling tree, exposing it to various fungal diseases, extracting material, and removing various branches to see what the effect would be on the tree—all invaluable insight for the farmer, he reasoned.

Later that day the farmer came out to check his fields and noticed the arborist conducting one of his experiments. He was unaware that the arborist was doing anything other than examining the trees and asked his friend what he was doing to the struggling tree. The arborist explained that he had been conducting experiments on the tree to learn how various conditions affect trees. He said that this information would help the survival and success of his remaining healthy trees. Seeing the value in this, the farmer nodded his head, indicating his approval of the continued experimentation. The experimentation provided useful data for the arborist, which determined why the tree had remained resilient for so long.

As the winter approached, workers used the arborist's recommendation to ensure that the trees were strong throughout the winter and would yield an even greater crop the following spring. The struggling tree, however, received none of the benefits of the data collected by the arborist because the tree had been written off as a lost cause. In fact, the tree was struggling to fight off a fungus that had been introduced by the arborist. The farmer was so happy that the healthy trees were blossoming that he failed to protest the treatment of the struggling tree and never considered that this tough tree, including the other three seeds that had prematurely died, could have survived and thrived had he only given it the attention and resources it needed and prevented the inequitable treatment it had endured from the arborist.

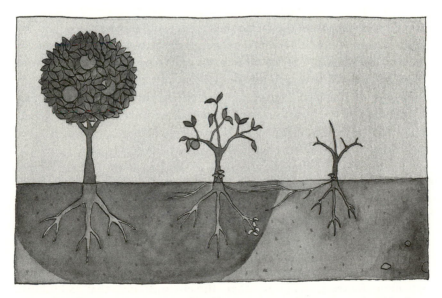

The impact of political determinants of health inequities on our ecosystem. Tim Kirby, from the collection of Daniel Dawes.

The End

Spring arrived, and the two trees in the rich soil were again strong and healthy. They produced their best fruit yet, and the farmer was overjoyed. However, the farmer and his workers arrived to a sad, yet foreseeable sight when they checked the poor soil. There in the midst of the land the struggling tree had succumbed to the neglectful conditions; the entire tree had fallen to the ground. Miraculously, it had grown large in spite of and, in some regards, in a defensive response to, the circumstances. The roots of the tree were thick but brittle, unable to hold the tree firmly in the ground. The branches were broad but weak, and there were no leaves or fruit. The trunk of the tree was covered in fungus and the inside had been hollowed out by bugs. The tree should have been magnificent, but now all that remained was a toppled shadow of what could have been.

The farmer and his workers surveyed his land. Surprisingly, they were well pleased with their progress and proud of their work. They beamed over the two surviving trees, notwithstanding that one tree had acquired a fungus when mycelium from the now dead tree in the poor soil had reached it, which made it less fruitful. These trees had been well cared for during all seasons of their lives. They would continue to produce a crop at a profit, and they would ensure the farmer had a relatively successful orchard for years to come. Only on a few rare occasions did he consider that he should have taken better care of the other seeds and trees, that with better care those trees would have also produced a crop at a profit, and that this increased profit would have ensured he had an even stronger and a more successful orchard for years to come. The farmer never considered the possibility that the tree he neglected might actually have been his strongest tree, as it somehow grew and produced fruit without adequate care.

Furthermore, no thought was given to the once beautiful then forgotten tree that had graced the horizon when the farmer originally arrived on the land. No one even spoke of it, of the ensuing problems it endured once it was uprooted and replanted in a less ideal part of the land. Not once did the farmer, his workers, or the arborist recognize that the orchard was indeed a pitiful sight, a graveyard of lost opportunities, a representation of a parochial view of success. The trees deserved appropriate attention and resources to overcome the circumstances that had limited their growth. A flourishing orchard could have been built around the existing tree. The depleted soils could have received additional treatment.

The ailing trees could have benefited from attention. The idea that there could have been seven healthy, strong, producing trees was somehow lost in the joy of the two trees that had so easily produced fruit owing to preferential treatment. The farmer had *an* orchard, but he did not achieve the orchard he could have had.

The Lesson

History is riddled with cautionary tales such as this one. Even the Bible recounts a similar story of mindlessly scattered and sown seeds and their unfortunate fate. The overarching moral of these stories warns us to take heed lest we follow the path of negligent farmers who were ultimately left with far less yield than they could have achieved had they taken proper care of their entire crops from beginning to end. The stories drive home the idea that improper planning, resources, care, and attention result in unfavorable outcomes, while proper care at the right time and in the right amount will encourage an endeavor to thrive.

The preceding parable is an allegory for the history of health inequities in the United States. It underscores the impact that political forces have on an individual's and the larger society's health and well-being: the political determinants of health. It highlights how inequities, when left unchecked, can sap a nation's strength. The allegory also reminds us to be cautious about the judgments we make about people because their health status is often based on their limited choices and opportunities. After all, regardless of our status, we all strive to improve our health and achieve health equity.

Since the founding of the United States of America, political forces have played a principal role in perpetuating and exacerbating health disparities at each stage of life—the beginning, the middle, and the end. The parable highlights the root causes of health inequities, with trees representing communities or people who can reach health equity (their optimal level of health), those who have died prematurely, and those who are barely hanging on to life. The allegory underscores how disparate treatment can hinder health and prematurely snuff out life.

In this story, the government is represented by the farmer, which at every stage of our life, whether through policy or legal actions or inactions, through a complex web of political structures and processes that have been created at the international, federal, state, and local levels, impacts our health status. The government either exacerbates health inequities or advances health equity for individuals or communities across the country. Like the farmer who failed to recognize the value and potential of all of his seeds and who failed to acknowledge or understand how his actions resulted in the loss of his crop, the government has oftentimes failed to take ownership for its actions or has been complicit with others, resulting in the outcomes we see today.

Native Americans, Alaska Natives, and Native Hawaiians have endured removal to reservations—some of the most brutal parts of the country—and today experience some of the highest health disparities in behavioral health and in systemic health. They, like the beautiful established tree encountered by the farmer when he arrived at the plot of land, were relocated and neglected by the government in pursuit of economic prosperity and security.

Similarly, the trees in the poor, rocky soil encompass other disparate groups, including lower socioeconomic status individuals, people with disabilities, racial and ethnic communities, lesbian, gay, bisexual, and transgender (LGBTQ+) individuals, veterans, children, women, immigrants, and older adults who have struggled to access quality education, gainful employment opportunities, safe and affordable housing, reliable transportation, and health care. Just as the seeds on the rocky and poor soil were neglected by the farmer, these groups struggle to attain better health outcomes and health equity owing to factors that often result directly from political action or inaction, which leads to disparate treatment and impact. For many people in these groups, health equity is not only out of reach, it is out of sight.

The Beginning

The allegory highlights the conditions and circumstances that plague our nation, including but not limited to generational and situational poverty; low standards of living; broken educational, criminal, and health systems; inadequate transportation; housing instability and insecurity; poor nutrition and diet; and lack of health literacy. In the allegory, the seed is the constant and the farmer and soil are the variables. Some of the farmer's seeds never had a chance. Just as he had done with the original majestic tree that he had removed from the nutrient-rich soil, the farmer placed them in less than ideal conditions and gave them insufficient resources and attention from the start. The seeds that *were* able to germinate, along with the majestic tree, continued to be plagued by the context of their circumstances and neglectful care, which began before the seeds even broke through the ground.

In this story, the soil represents housing, a crucial but underestimated factor affecting health. As researchers have found, "residential segregation remains a root cause of racial disparities in health today."[2] The depth of each hole, the careless placement of the seeds in the poor and rocky soils, and the environmental conditions these seeds found themselves represent the structural barriers that must be overcome, including racism, implicit bias, and other forms of unjustified discrimination manifested in racially restrictive covenants, mortgage loans redlining, and unfavorable property appraisals. When the strong wind blows the seed away that is aboveground or torrential rain washes the seed away or the sun bakes the seed, these create the barriers that detrimentally affect the seeds.

The fertilizer represents education and underscores the inequitable delivery of education by the government based on a system that rewards more affluent communities. The water represents economic or employment opportunities enabled or stifled by the government. The pesticide represents health care as a preventive measure or treatment for health conditions, and highlights the disproportionate availability and delivery of health services that depend on your zip code, including medical, mental health, oral health, and public health. The care or lack thereof that the farmer showed each tree during its life span represents the government's neglect, which leads to many voiceless communities experiencing increased mental health and substance use challenges. Furthermore, the investments that the farmer refused to give the tree in the poor soil represent the lack of funding for social or human services intended to bolster social and economic opportunities for underresourced communities.

Environmental determinants of health in certain geographic and demographic contexts aggravate these issues. Such effects have resulted in toxic sites; substandard plumbing; polluted air, waters, and lands; and insufficient access to fresh and nutritious foods. Because of political determinants, population groups have been pushed into geographic areas unsuitable for sustaining life, resulting in significant and lasting impact on their health and well-being. Studies have shown that zip code more than genetic code predicts your health status and life expectancy. Where you work, live, sleep, eat, learn, pray, and play significantly impact your overall health status. Many people are aware of the historic divide between northern and southern states in the United States. However, fewer people are aware of the health and health care implications between the North and South. The South has the highest chronic disease rates and disparities in health status in the country among racial and ethnic groups, giving it the unenviable title as the diabetes belt, heart disease belt, and cancer belt of America. While the North has achieved higher-quality health care and lower chronic disease rates, it, too, has had challenges ensuring that higher-quality health care translates to all communities regardless of socioeconomic status, race, or ethnicity.

Rural populations across the country have long struggled to obtain primary care and hospital services. Depending on their geographic location, they may even experience disproportionate rates of chronic diseases or higher burden from behavioral health risks. For instance, rural communities in the South have long experienced higher rates of poverty, smoking, physical inactivity, and death due to heart disease and diabetes; rural communities in the West have higher rates of alcohol misuse and suicide; and rural communities in the Northeast have higher rates of total tooth loss.[3]

There are also considerable disparities in health status and health care among other underserved populations. Members of racial and ethnic minority groups experience higher mortality rates and earlier onset of diseases. They also receive lower-quality health care, leading to worse health care outcomes. African American women have the highest death rates from heart disease, breast and lung cancer, stroke, and pregnancy among women of all racial and ethnic backgrounds. Hispanics have poorer quality of care than non-Hispanic whites for about 40 percent of quality measures, including not receiving screening for cancer or cardiovascular risk factors. American Indians and Alaska Natives have a suicide rate that is 50 percent higher than the national average, and Asian Americans have a high prevalence of chronic obstructive pulmonary disease, hepatitis B, tuberculosis, and liver disease.[4]

In general, people with disabilities are more likely to have difficulty or experience delays in accessing vital health services, including oral health care. Individuals with serious mental illness die on average twenty-five years earlier than the general population, at age fifty-three. LGBTQ+ individuals also experience a disproportionate burden from discrimination and disease. They are approximately two-and-a-half times more likely than heterosexuals to have a mental health disorder in their lifetime, and studies have shown that discrimination against LGBTQ+ persons has been associated with high rates of depression, substance use, and suicide.[5]

The lack of attention given to the various soils at planting symbolizes the extent to which some people, before they are born, are denied the firm foundation needed to obtain optimal health. Before life begins, with the prenatal health of the mother, you can see the effects of geographic and circumstantial context in human lives, and the vicious cycle perpetuated when the government fails to intervene and provide an equitable solution or intervenes by enacting policies that create, preserve, or exacerbate the inequities. Rather than understanding and addressing the context in which people are born or placed, the political system often fails to overcome structural and procedural barriers to provide the necessary support and resources people need to have adequate access and availability to quality education, jobs, health care, behavioral health services, and social services.

As a society, we have been conditioned to believe that *equality*, which is giving everyone the same treatment, is the solution for all. When, in fact, *equity*, which is rooted in the principle of distributive justice or "concern with the apportionment of privileges, duties, and goods in consonance with the merits of the individual and in the best interest of society,"[6] is what society should be striving for. Opportunities equally distributed do not address the individual needs and circumstances of a community. The notion of equality fails to appreciate the multidimensional systemic issues involving economic, social, cultural, historical, and political factors that unfairly advantage some groups and disadvantage others. From the beginning, the trees in the poor soil and the rocky area of the land were structurally disadvantaged, while the trees in the nutrient-rich soil were structurally advantaged. Even if the farmer and his workers had employed a one-size-fits-all approach and given each tree the same treatment, such as the same amount of fertilizer, water, sunshine, or pesticides, it would not have been enough to help each tree reach its optimal level of health because the farmer and his workers failed to address the root causes of the problem—allocating the necessary resources and attention each tree needed, depending on its circumstances.

The Middle

The farmer should have analyzed the soil before planting the seeds and nourished the soil accordingly. He should have thought more seriously about his larger vision of establishing a flourishing orchard and treated his seeds equitably, giving them what they needed, when they needed it, and in the amount they needed to reach their optimal health. These efforts are important for a thriving community where people are able to reach their full potential and contribute to the benefit of society.

If the farmer aimed to produce the best crop, he should have removed some of the stones from the rocky soil and brought in additional soil. He should have added additional fertilizer and watered the seeds in the poor soil. If he sought to have the strongest trees, he should have intervened early, examined the struggling tree, identified the source of the disease, and found solutions to eliminate the problems. The key to understanding equitable treatment is that the attention given to the needs of the seeds in the poor and rocky soils does not take away from the needs of the seeds in the nutrient-rich soil. Providing for the individual needs of the seeds within their respective soils would have given him more trees, more crops, and more prosperity, allowing each tree to be healthy, just as a healthier and more productive citizenry would lead to a stronger democracy and cost savings for the government.

For more than 225 years, the United States has struggled with aligning the constitutional notions of equal protection and general welfare to our laws and policies. We saw this in segregated schools and hospitals, in our criminal justice system, and with legal discrimination in housing. Historically, the United States has failed to recognize that achieving health equity requires valuing each group equally and recognizing their contributions. The farmer valued the seeds he planted in the rich soil more than he valued the seeds he planted in the poor and rocky soil, as evidenced by his placement of the seeds in suboptimal areas and the inequitable distribution of resources and attention he afforded the trees in the nutrient-rich soil. The seeds in the rich soil were given additional resources considerably beyond what they needed to reach their full potential, while the seeds in the rocky and poor soil were not given the additional resources they needed to develop and thrive. In many respects, our political system has demonstrated intentional and unintentional biases that favor one group versus others, even when they are suffering from the same ailments, such as HIV/AIDS, opioid addiction, and mental illness. These biases are evidenced by developing and executing policies that have punished one group or protected another group for the same offenses or neglecting or withholding resources from a less valued group with little or no power and privilege. From the point of conception to birth and beyond, we can see the effects of policy on various groups creating a vicious cycle of inequities fueled by personal, economic, and security interests.

As the trees in our allegory grew, the farmer failed to recognize that targeted care was required at this point because the trees had not started from the same place or been given the same amount of care and treatment. The farmer did not treat all the trees the same because he made some judgments about their likelihood of success owing to the soil they were planted in and therefore treated them differently. The two "bad soil seed" groups were treated more alike than the "good soil seeds." In many respects, individuals deemed as bad seeds are blamed for their circumstances and prejudged about their likelihood to succeed based on various social factors, including their zip code. Those deemed as bad seeds, such as people of color, are grouped together and treated similarly (discriminated against) because of their difference from the good seeds (the privileged), again based on prejudice.

Even when the farmer decided to give his vulnerable tree extra fertilizer and the workers irrigated the tree's roots, they failed to appreciate the extent of the problem or what resources and how much would be needed to help the tree reach its full potential. Even when something is done to address the problem, it is sometimes done because of how it affects the majority (who is the priority) and not necessarily for the betterment of the affected population. Consequentially, this story highlights that there are often unnoticeable political determinants throughout our nation's history built on underlying structural racism, misogyny, and other forms of unconscionable discrimination.

Sometimes extemporaneous interceding factors also severely impact our health and well-being and may result in the premature death of individuals and communities. The storm that represents the brutal forces that roll in unexpectedly and cut your life short, such as violence or natural disasters—the effects of which can be mitigated or worsened by political systems—illustrate this point. Examples of interceding factors could be seen in the failure of the federal government to adequately respond to the aftermaths of Hurricane Katrina, which devastated New Orleans, Louisiana, and Hurricane Maria, which devastated Puerto Rico and the US Virgin Islands, both United States territories. In contrast, the political response to Hurricane Michael, which devastated Florida and Georgia, and Hurricane Harvey, which devastated Houston, Texas, was significantly different because those communities were valued differently. While the forces that created these disasters were natural, the severity and disproportionality of their impact were, in effect, unnatural disasters, or environmental injustices, owing to political determinants that were built on underlying structural racism and other forms of discrimination.

Finally, the farmer made insufficient attempts to comprehensively assess and diagnose the problems impacting each tree and authorize the necessary treatment plan so that each tree stood a fair chance of obtaining its full potential. Rather than conduct a thorough assessment of the tree to correctly determine the source of the problem (which, in this case, was signified by the bugs gnawing at the roots of the tree in the poor, sandy soil), the farmer became absorbed with other issues—oblivious to the main problem—and thus instituted piecemeal or short-sighted approaches to address the superficial problems plaguing the trees in the poor, sandy soil and poor, rocky soil.

Similarly, our health system has failed to treat the whole problem—addressing the seen and unseen factors impacting health and wellness—including the behavioral, social, and environmental determinants of health but most important, for the purposes of this discussion, the political determinants of health. The disease within the tree (insidious yet powerful determinants not always obvious or prioritized because they are frequently blamed on the individual instead of the disease nature of the issues or the environmental factors that exacerbate the problem) represents the challenges to recognizing the impact of behavioral health or oral health on systemic health. They are equally important to your overall health, but it has been difficult to prioritize policies and allocate resources, elevating them on par with less stigmatized diseases. To change the trajectory of these seeds, or groups, that endure inequities, real change must take place at the deepest level to have lasting and meaningful impact. It requires thoughtfully assessing a problem all the way down to the subterranean level to better understand the root causes of the problems to develop more effective solutions.

The sick tree was subjected to the experimentation of an arborist who should have been caring for the tree or at least trying to assess the cause of the tree's problems. Instead, with the farmer's consent, he used the sick yet resilient tree as a specimen to glean valuable information to benefit other trees. In this allegory, the arborist represents both private individuals and groups that have leveraged the political system to further their unscrupulous or profit-driven agendas without regard to the effect on the individuals experimented on. This same concept is borne out historically. Experiments on vulnerable groups and subjugating groups to disparate treatment are well documented.[7] Although the government has engaged in experiments on certain population groups, the arborist's experimentations on the weak tree represent a system's complicity in research conducted by nongovernmental parties on unwitting African Americans,[8] Native Americans, Puerto Ricans, low-income individuals, incarcerated individuals,[9] children in foster care, and people with disabilities.[10]

Specifically, black women, Native American women, Puerto Rican women, and women with mental illnesses were subjected to gynecological experiments in the past. More recently, in the last few decades, experiments were conducted on other vulnerable populations. Hundreds of black men, part of an infamous syphilis observational study from 1932 to 1972, who were suffering from syphilis were left untreated without their consent. In the 1950s and 1960s, vulnerable children and youth with developmental disabilities were experimented on with radioactive milk and with hepatitis. As recently as 2004, news broke about the use of children in foster care in AIDS drugs experiments. In the 1970s, most pharmaceutical experiments were conducted on incarcerated individuals to study everything from chemical warfare agents to testing dandruff treatments. The United States also engaged in syphilis experiments outside the country on Guatemalan prisoners in 1946. Perpetrators have included clinicians, researchers, scientists, lawyers, administrators, entrepreneurs, and other professionals as well as corporations and other organizations that have worked with or solicited the government's approval for their conduct.

The arborist and the farmer later used the valuable data they gleaned from the experiments to "help" protect and strengthen the livelihood of the other more healthy trees. In a similar vein, data collected from disenfranchised groups have been used in the United States against them for purposes of "protecting" or enhancing services to more privileged groups. One such troubling episode involves the government's census data, which was used in the past to target specific populations. According to reports, the collected data from the 1940 Census "was secretly used in one of the worst violations of constitutional rights in U.S. history: the internment of Japanese Americans during World War II." A year before, in 1939, the Federal Bureau of Investigation along with military intelligence agencies joined forces to "relax census confidentiality rules in the hope of accessing data on individuals. However, the effort was opposed by Census Bureau Director William Lane Austin." After refusing to relax the census confidentiality rules, the Census Bureau director was forced to retire once the 1940 presidential election was over. Austin's replacement did not share the former director's position on confidentiality and immediately went to work to remove those rules, which eventually cleared the way for other governmental agencies to access the information on Japanese Americans.[11]

The fungi represent the insidious and lingering effects of structural racism, misogyny, homophobia, ableism, and other treacherous forms of inequality undergirding the political determinants of health, which has affected various groups for generations. It highlights the stain of slavery, racial segregation, and unjustified discrimination against racial and ethnic groups, people with disabilities, people with mental illness and substance use disorders, LGBTQ+ individuals, and others. When it was over, the farmer had trees only where he had invested his time and resources. The other trees succumbed to external pressures exacerbated by the actions of the farmer and the arborist.

Advocates in partnership with policy makers have historically championed causes that would bolster health equity, moving the nation a few steps closer to reaching this audacious goal, but once the political winds shifted, advocates have found themselves losing some of those steps, unable to stop the political pendulum from swinging too far back and unraveling the gains that took generations to achieve, as documented in my book *150 Years of ObamaCare*. Just as the soil served as a foundation or determinant for each tree's future health status, the political environment and the strength of advocacy efforts have consistently determined the success of each policy attempt to elevate health equity in America. It should be troubling that some groups of people are born into this world confronting obstacles, barriers, and disparities, which prevent them from reaching a "state of complete physical, mental and social well-being."[12] It should be troubling that some groups of people confront obstacles, barriers, and disparities to their end-of-life care that prevent them from dying with dignity, facing unfair treatment until their last breath.

Conclusion

History is replete with examples of political systems ignoring the voice of justice. In some instances, the political determinants have elevated efforts to advance health equity for all groups, but on more occasions, they have hindered the advancement of health equity. Political strategies, decisions, and actions have resulted in reinforcing systems that ensure the status quo or dismantling systems that challenge the status quo. As we seed the ground and move forward on this journey to health equity, it is important to understand what has caused portions of the field to become barren so we can fertilize the soil to promote political action on health equity.

The moral of the story underscores the notion that if you think that you are immune from what happens to others, you are sadly mistaken. As Professor Suzanne Simard's research on trees has shown, trees talk with and provide nutrients to one another, which ensure the overall health of the forest. As with trees, humans are interconnected. Political systems at all levels should take note that the lives of its citizens are inextricably intertwined and that, when one community is negatively affected, other communities will also be negatively impacted. As the allegory of the orchard proves, society is only going to be as strong as its foundation and its fortitude to address the political determinants of health. What follows is intended to strengthen this foundation and galvanize our commitment to tackling the political determinants of health.

This book proceeds in six parts. Chapter 2 recounts and examines specific efforts to leverage political determinants to address and rectify health inequities in America. Chapter 3 defines and discusses the political determinants of health and provides a new framework from which to analyze the barriers and interventions in achieving health equity in the United States and beyond. Chapters 4 and 5 demonstrate how the political determinants of health recently led to greater prioritization of health equity at the federal level, laying out in great detail the strategies and tactics that enabled the most inclusive health policy to be developed, passed, and implemented in the United States. Chapter 6 discusses oppositional efforts to undermine health equity-focused policies and how health equity leaders have been tackling the political determinants of health inequities during a challenging period. Chapter 7 discusses future political challenges to health equity and provides readers with an example of how the political determinants of health model may be used to elevate health equity.

2

Setting the Precedent

America's Attempts to Address the Political Determinants of Health Inequities

They were enslaved by law, emancipated by law, disenfranchised and segregated by law; and, finally, they have begun to win equality by law. Along the way, new constitutional principles have emerged to meet the challenges of a changing society. The progress has been dramatic, and it will continue.—*Thurgood Marshall, US Supreme Court Justice, "The Bicentennial Speech"*

Many people are familiar with the movement to increase access to health care and treatments in the United States, but fewer people are aware that underlying that movement has been another one intended to expose and unravel the inequities in health status and health care that aggregate over time and impact the entire life course. This health equity movement has been working tirelessly to stretch the umbrella of inclusivity just a little bit wider so that the gains made by the larger movement would benefit as many groups as possible. The goal has long been to create a more healthy, equitable, and inclusive society.

The history of health equity advocacy in the United States reveals a pattern of political determinants rooted in the nation's founding and inscribed in its Constitution: conflicts among the branches of the federal government and between the federal and state governments over the power to offer and fund programs to bolster the welfare of its citizens; endemic and ongoing polarization between two political parties, resulting in pendulum swings in health policies; persistent divisions stemming from the nation's slaveholding past that have consistently disadvantaged racial and other minority populations; capitalist biases that promote commerce over economic equity to the ongoing detriment of the underprivileged. These political determinants of health are the main drivers of inequities in America but the least understood.

If health equity is the absence of avoidable or remediable differences in health among groups of people,[1] then, conversely, health inequities in our society are not the result of the natural order of things, which means there is something we can actually do about them. Health inequities are, instead, owing to a history of political and legal precedent that have baked into our systems the discriminatory standards, practices, and beliefs we observe or experience today. They reinforce existing policies and influence new policies. This unequal treatment has resulted in inequities in health, education, employment, housing, criminal justice, transportation, and a host of other variables that collectively affect our ability to attain outstanding health outcomes, to achieve higher life expectancies, and to ensure the opportunity for all groups living in the United States to meaningfully contribute to strengthening our democracy.

Proponents of health equity need to recognize these systemic political obstacles. They must also learn from those who have successfully bypassed or overcome these obstacles by leveraging the electoral process to install elected officials committed to health equity, by crafting persuasive arguments that underscore the economic and national security benefits of enhanced health outcomes, and by acting with persistence and urgency. Most important, health equity proponents must learn how previous champions united their independent efforts to overcome the intrapersonal, interpersonal, institutional, and structural barriers that have prevented us from reaching underserved populations and elevating health equity for all groups. The following provides an overview of the attempts to address health inequities in the United States by leveraging the interventions of the political determinants of health.

The First Attempt: Recruiting America's Most Prominent Health Equity Leader

In 1775, before the United States of America existed, a group of advocates organized in Pennsylvania for the purpose of not only abolishing slavery in colonial America but also integrating freed slaves in society. One year later, during the American Revolutionary War, the advocates realized some success by increasing national attention and discourse on the inherent rights of people and gained support for their argument that the slave trade was an abomination and should be ended.[2] So effective were these advocates, that even Thomas Jefferson while drafting the Declaration of Independence, inserted a passage "blaming King George III for the transatlantic slave trade," and declaring that the King of England had quashed legislative attempts to abolish it, but John Adams and Benjamin Franklin struck it, believing that it would have been too controversial.[3]

Immediately following the end of the American Revolutionary War in 1784, the advocates regrouped in Pennsylvania "'for promoting the abolition of slavery, and the relief of free negroes, unlawfully held in [b]ondage, and for [i]mproving the [c]ondition of the African [r]ace.'"[4] The next year, Alexander Hamilton in conjunction with John Jay organized a similar initiative in New York. Collectively, this movement to abolish slavery and address enslaved people's welfare picked up greater steam in the ensuing years and resulted in strategic advocacy efforts to inform the fledgling nation about the evils of slavery. It was an issue that abolitionists tirelessly advocated for during the constitutional debates, which resulted in a compromise that would not offend either the North or the South once the Constitution of the United States was signed in 1787.[5]

In 1789, the US Congress formally convened. As the first Congress was getting settled and figuring out how to govern, the advocates met regularly to strategize and build consensus around a plan of action to abolish slavery and afford enslaved people and other vulnerable populations access to resources and services to improve their health and reach their optimal level of health. They enlisted the help of one of America's most prolific and gifted politicos, Benjamin Franklin. Although a former slave owner himself, Franklin had allowed the publication of articles in his newspapers decrying slavery, and as he matured, he came to view slavery as an evil institution. Advocates pleaded with Franklin to use his platform and influence to urge his friends and colleagues, now part of the newly established government, to address this institutionalized immorality. Franklin gave in, and, during the second year of the first Congress, he decided to act.

Franklin sent a petition[6] dated February 3, 1790, to the leaders of the newly formed US Congress, the president of the Senate, and the Speaker of the House, urging them to end the institution of slavery in the United States and promote mercy and justice toward enslaved individuals. Within this petition was the first grassroots attempt to essentially address the social determinants of health and advance health equity for all population groups by doing everything possible to promote the general welfare of all "descriptions of people" residing in the country. He argued that the newly established Congress had powers vested in them to "promot[e] the welfare and secur[e] the blessings of liberty to the people of the United States, without distinction of color, to all descriptions of people" and urged "that nothing, which can be done for the relief of the unhappy objects of their care, will be either omitted or delayed."[7]

The petition was introduced to the House on February 12, 1790, and three days later in the Senate. Highly contentious, it resulted in fiery debates in both chambers, leading proslavery members of Congress to denounce it.[8] In a formal report on March 5, 1790, less than one month after receiving Franklin's petition, Congress responded, arguing that the Constitution rendered it powerless to do anything to help those already enslaved on US soil, much less provide access to health care for these vulnerable populations. The congressional report explicitly argued that the federal government had no authority to address the general welfare of enslaved individuals and tackle what we now refer to as the social determinants of health.

The first Congress was concerned about the effect that Franklin's petition would have on the young democracy and opined that it had "no authority to interfere in the internal regulations of particular states"[9] relative to ensuring adequate clothing, accommodations, and subsistence; preventing the separation of children from their parents; and ensuring a comfortable provision in cases of sickness, age, or infirmity. Of course, the balance between federalism (a stronger federal government) and confederalism (a weaker federal government) was not a settled issue at this point, nor is it now, but throughout US history, federalism has been endorsed when it serves the party in power and when there is an attempt to prioritize health equity nationally. The first Congress's decision was a lost opportunity to advance health equity for all Americans and a blow to the advocates who had worked tirelessly to plead their case for the creation of policies that would afford "all descriptions of people" living in the country a fair opportunity for happiness.

John Adams, as vice president under George Washington and president of the Senate, received Franklin's petition, but he too bowed to pressure from slavery proponents concerned about upsetting the new and fragile republic. Franklin died several weeks after Congress formally responded to his petition. Surprisingly, just eight years later, in 1798, Congress passed the first significant federal health care legislation[10] into law when John Adams succeeded George Washington as president. This health policy was developed by Congress to provide relief to sick and disabled sailors, ignoring its earlier declaration that it was powerless to create and enforce policies tackling access to health care and the social determinants of health owing to a confederalism argument that it did not have the "authority to interfere in the internal regulations of particular states."

The 1798 legislation—An Act for the Relief of Sick and Disabled Seamen—created the Marine Hospital Service and mandated that privately employed sailors purchase health insurance. Merchant marines often got injured or contracted tropical diseases, leaving captains without enough sailors to operate, putting a strain on the nation's economy. Realizing that a healthy maritime workforce was essential to the ability of merchant ships to facilitate commerce, Congress and the president resolved to do something about it.

The Marine Hospital Service consisted of a series of hospitals built and operated by the federal government to treat privately employed sailors. This service was financed by a mandatory tax on each maritime sailor's income that was to be paid by the owner or captain of each vessel. This tax equated to twenty cents per sailor for each month of employment. On passage of the law, ships were no longer permitted to sail in and out of US ports unless the health care tax had been collected by shipowners and paid to the government. When sailors needed medical assistance, the government would confirm that their payments had been collected and then give them a voucher to be admitted to the treating hospital. The system was eventually expanded to cover sailors working private vessels on the Mississippi and Ohio Rivers. This program eventually became the Public Health Service.

Policy reflects the values of its time. Note that the early government interceded and exercised its power to promote the general welfare in the provision of health care, depending on who was impacted—not for slaves but for sailors. It acted quickly for a certain group when it was perceived that there was a direct threat to commerce. The early government was restrained in applying the notion of equality across all population groups and was quick to shoot down any intervention relative to health care for powerless and underprivileged groups when it was perceived that the policy would negatively impact commerce. But it failed to understand that the health and well-being of everyone within its jurisdiction affected the economy and national security.

The Second Attempt: Passing America's First Health Equity-Focused Law

More than fifty years after Congress refused to embrace its power to extend health care rights to vulnerable groups, social reformers intent on advancing mental health and minority health reforms realized some progress in leveraging the political determinants. The mid-1800s saw the first successful legislation in Congress that addressed the social determinants of health for a broad swath of the US population, including housing, clothing, food, education, employment, and security. Before this, the primary reason a slave's health would come up in the law was when lawsuits were filed by disgruntled buyers of slaves complaining "that the slave was sick, or mentally ill, or a runaway, and that the owner had known about this fact, and cheated the buyer." Interestingly, "these cases were, in fact, the most common of all civil cases involving slaves, throughout the South."[11] However, even with the successful passage and enactment of the United States' first legislation addressing the social determinants of health, this remarkable policy accomplishment was short-lived because the statute was later wiped out by a president and a Congress determined to repeal it. Later civil rights laws would also be short-lived when they came before the US Supreme Court. For both mental health and minority health advocacy groups, it would take almost a century to achieve noteworthy, yet piecemeal, gains in federal policy.

Advocates for mental health, minority health, and other causes labored tirelessly to develop, introduce, pass, and implement legislation intended to benefit their own respective groups. They often advocated independently for their own priorities, employing autonomous campaigns and strategies and were met with limited progress. When one group successfully lobbied for its priorities, another group found itself on the losing end of the fight.

In the early 1800s, Dorothea Dix, a schoolteacher from Cambridge, Massachusetts, was inspired to take up the cause of those with mental health challenges and dedicated her time to changing public consciousness about these issues. This was not an easy feat, given that, according to Dr. King Davis, one of the nation's most accomplished mental health scholars, "some policymakers saw blacks as immune from mental illness, along with poor whites, women and Indians because they lacked the ability to reason."[12] Dix highlighted the abuses against prisoners and individuals with mental illness, including the intentional beating, starvation, chaining, and physical and sexual abuse of people with mental health conditions. She spent years traveling to several states sounding the alarm about the inhumane conditions people with mental illnesses were subjected to and urged legislatures to provide adequate institutions to treat and care for these individuals.

In the course of this work, Dix had learned that many states were unable or unwilling to bear the cost of these institutions; she decided then to turn to the federal government to provide aid. In 1848, she urged Congress to authorize a grant of five million acres of public lands, which would be sold and the proceeds used "as a perpetual fund for the care of the indigent insane." She believed that Congress might provide the grants, as they had previously done so to build roads, enhance public education, and make other domestic improvements. However, no action was taken on the proposal.[13]

In 1850, Dix again brought forward her proposal, this time requesting ten million acres of land. Debate on the bill aired conflicting views about how federal public lands should be used, with little to no attention paid to the needs of people with mental illness. Only Senator William Dawson of Georgia argued for the bill's humanitarian intent: "We cannot do a more charitable act than that which is proposed by this bill." The bill passed in the Senate but was deferred in the House. Dix advocated for the bill again in 1852, but no action was taken in either chamber of Congress. Finally, in 1854, Dix successfully lobbied for the Bill for the Benefit of the Indigent Insane, after having succeeded in various states by acquiring state funding to increase mental health care services. She had done so after developing reports on substandard mental health care for each state she visited, which led to the creation and passage of bills to establish psychiatric facilities. The congressional Bill for the Benefit of the Indigent Insane finally passed the Senate and the House and was sent to President Franklin Pierce to be signed into law.[14]

Dix and other mental health advocates were ecstatic. They believed that the political stars had finally aligned and that President Pierce would surely sign the mental health reform bill into law since he had witnessed a tragic train accident that horrifically killed his own son and resulted in his wife's severe bouts of depression and anxiety. The president himself became a substance misuser—an alcoholic. Nevertheless, the brief period of elation advocates enjoyed ended when Pierce vetoed the legislation and quashed the dreams and hopes of health equity champions. Pierce believed that it would be unconstitutional to regard health as anything but a private, nongovernmental matter. He argued:

> I readily and, I trust, feelingly acknowledge the duty incumbent on us all as men and citizens, and as among the highest and holiest of our duties, to provide for those who, in the mysterious order of Providence, are subject to

want and to disease of body or mind; but I cannot find any authority in the Constitution for making the Federal Government the great almoner of public charity throughout the United States. To do so would, in my judgment, be contrary to the letter and spirit of the Constitution and subversive of the whole theory upon which the Union of these States is founded.[15]

Pierce's veto set the policy of extremely limited federal participation or nonparticipation in the realm of mental health and social welfare for almost the next one hundred years. This essentially resulted in more direct advocacy at the state level where advocates initiated ballot measures and advocated for policies to advance mental health reforms after efforts at the federal level died. In this case, instead of the argument over federal powers versus states' rights, a tug-of-war between state and local governments erupted over who should assume responsibility and pay for mental health reforms. Most states assumed responsibility for mental health care by building and operating asylums, and local governments paid for episodic care.

Seven years after Dorothea Dix and other mental health reformers attempted to pass mental health reforms in the United States, the Civil War intervened. Before the Civil War ended in 1863, abolitionists had advocated, through petitions and direct lobbying, for a bureau that would provide protection, support, and access to health care, education, and employment for newly freed people. After the legislation was introduced, the House spent two months debating it and narrowly passed it by a vote of 69-67. The bill was then referred to the Senate's Select Committee on Slavery and Freedom where debate centered on which federal department should manage the proposed bureau: the Department of the Treasury or the Department of War. The original House bill had placed the proposed bureau in the Department of War, but the Senate changed the language to place it in the Department of the Treasury. The Senate passed its amended Freedmen's Bureau bill on June 28, 1864, by a vote of 21-9, but the House would not agree to the change, which meant that both chambers of Congress had to go to conference.

During debates in the conference committee, congressional members produced a new bill on February 2, 1865. This new bill only caused more heated debate about the federal government's role in providing special treatment to one group of people at the exclusion of another group and led to a demand for a second conference committee. It ultimately reverted to the House's original proposal to place the bureau in the Department of

War. Notwithstanding a significant number of senators remaining opposed to the legislation, the Senate finally adopted the conference report on March 3, 1865, by a vote of 21-9, with 22 abstentions.[16]

While abolitionists continued to press their advocacy agenda for the bureau, a public health threat helped the bill get over the finish line. After the Civil War, when slaves were emancipated and moved into cities in large numbers, a health crisis occurred that required the federal government's involvement. Even with this health crisis, Congress could only secure the votes to pass a bill providing most of the necessities of life, but they could not convince the majority of congressional lawmakers to retain language authorizing the bureau to provide health care to former slaves. Despite the heroic attempts by abolitionists to include specific language pertaining to access to medical care, lawmakers struck the language during negotiations involving the Freedmen's Bureau Act.

In the spirit of compromise, Congress grudgingly approved the creation of the Freedmen's Bureau without the health care provision. It became formally known as the Bureau of Refugees, Freedmen and Abandoned Lands. Ironically, to pass a bill that would benefit individuals who had formerly been enslaved, congressional sympathizers had to include language supportive of former Confederate soldiers displaced as a result of the war. There simply was no appetite to pass legislation that would solely benefit freed people or former slaves who were not yet considered full citizens. Moving forward, any federal legislation that was enacted into law in the United States to bolster minority health was only successful if it included provisions to elevate the health status of lower-socioeconomic-status whites, too. The Freedmen's Bureau was a federal agency that aided former slaves during the post–Civil War Reconstruction era. Its purpose was to provide food and emergency relief to freed people and poor whites in war-torn areas, to regulate the labor of the freed people, to administer justice, to manage land confiscated during the war, and to establish schools for the freed people.

One month after the legislation was signed into law, President Abraham Lincoln was assassinated. After his death, as the policy was being implemented, Lincoln's supporters argued they had the authority to provide health care to freed people and refugees under the new program, even though the statute contained no provisions for medical care. During slavery, although the provision of medical care to sick slaves was a last resort, there was a profit motive to keep slaves healthy, but after the Civil War, doctors and hospitals refused to provide medical care to black people.[17] Andrew Johnson,[18] who had assumed the presidency following Lincoln's assassination, vetoed a bill intended to increase the power of the Freedmen's Bureau in the beginning of 1866. In his veto message, he used the arguments of congressional opponents of the measure, namely, "it was unnecessary to extend the original legislation, it infringed on states' rights, it gave the federal government an unprecedented role in providing aid to a specific group of people at the exclusion of others, and it was expensive."[19]

The bill Johnson had vetoed in early 1866 was subsequently reintroduced, scaled back, and passed by Congress in the summer of 1866 along with another major bill, the Civil Rights Act of 1866. Again Johnson vetoed both bills, but proponents of the measures succeeded in garnering enough votes to overturn his veto.

During the congressional elections that fall, Johnson toured the nation, stumping for individuals more closely aligned with his policy agenda, but abolitionists were successful in getting more people who were aligned with their cause elected to the House and Senate, which effectively gave Republicans a two-thirds majority in both chambers as well as in state legislatures in the North.[20] This allowed Lincoln's supporters to continue their Reconstruction and civil rights agenda and ensured that efforts to address the social determinants of health would be implemented.[21]

Congress reauthorized the Freedmen's Bureau every year until 1869, one year after the Fourteenth Amendment to the Constitution was ratified, declaring all former slaves US citizens.[22] At every chance, opponents of health equity sought to use the elections to highlight their policy agenda. In 1866, the American citizenry rejected efforts to undermine Reconstruction and civil rights, but during the 1868 presidential election, opponents of health equity started to effectively mobilize, running on a platform of voiding reconstruction. During this time, six former Confederate states— Alabama, Florida, Georgia, Louisiana, North Carolina, and South Carolina— were readmitted to the Union, and, from that time onward, opponents of health equity successfully captured congressional seats in elections.[23]

The readmission of former confederate states bolstered opponents' efforts to leverage the political determinants in preventing health equity initiatives. However, proponents of health equity also leveraged political determinants and worked diligently to register approximately seven hundred three thousand African Americans to vote the year before.[24] Ulysses Grant won the presidential election on a platform of peace and unity, but his victory was narrow. He won by a little over three hundred thousand votes, a victory attributed to the five hundred thousand votes of newly enfranchised black voters.[25]

Following his election, the Freedmen's Bureau created and funded a medical division to address the health care needs of the newly freed slaves, which by 1870 had numbered almost five million people.[26] The bureau established hospitals and dispensaries throughout the South, for the most part using existing buildings, such as abandoned mansions. The bureau's doctors also provided home visits, through which patients with less acute illnesses could receive care. During the fewer than seven years of the Freedmen's Bureau's existence, the medical division established more than ninety hospitals and other health facilities throughout the South, providing care to well over five hundred thousand patients, or nearly 10 percent of the black population. The facilities, however, suffered from insufficient funding, supplies, and staff. The bureau often struggled with recruiting physicians, nurses, and other health professionals, and the health professionals it recruited were frequently inexperienced or unqualified. Conditions in some of the hospitals were so unsanitary that they resulted in illnesses and deaths, for the bureau lacked funds to address this issue, much less buy proper food for patients.

While the Freedmen's Bureau was in operation, the political determinants played a major role in undermining not only its success but also the success of other government-initiated programs. The federal government had chartered the Freedmen's Savings and Trust Company, where many newly freed people invested their savings. When white executives, who were responsible for managing the freedmen's bank, made poor investment choices, legislators and regulators would not step in. Instead, they allowed market forces to discriminate against the newly freed people. This would not be the only time in US history that the government allowed this to happen. The government enabled economic discrimination to recur well into the future. In the 1930s, the Home Owners' Loan Corporation, established under President Franklin D. Roosevelt's New Deal, engaged in redlining communities and denying mortgages to communities of color, immigrant communities, and other communities graded poorly by this government-sponsored program.[27]

Congress voted to completely shut down the Freedmen's Bureau in June 1872, after barely seven years of operation. Although it fell short of providing adequate necessities, security, and quality health care to millions of former slaves, the bureau was not shuttered for its performance but owing to racial politics. Congress's decision to terminate the Freedmen's Bureau stands as perhaps the only time Congress effectively dismantled a major federal statutorily authorized program focused on addressing the social determinants of health. The bureau's closing would be felt by generations of African American and poor white families for almost a century and a half. Millions of vulnerable communities would find themselves unable to access care and treatment when they needed it most. In the era of Jim Crow laws, between 1877 to the mid-1960s, many hospitals and other health care facilities refused to provide care or lifesaving treatments to African Americans.

The Third Attempt: The Great Awakening and Disappointment for Health Equity

Almost one hundred years after the first major attempt to pass comprehensive mental health reform legislation in the United States under President Pierce, advocates reengaged in the political process once Harry Truman was elected president following World War II. The war had exposed serious health issues among Americans, including high rates of malnutrition and unaddressed mental health issues. It had also exposed the dangers of racial discrimination in the military. Health equity proponents hoped, at long last, that Truman would be the president who would usher in health reforms, including mental health reforms. As with the election of Lincoln, the political system allowed a fundamental shift in health policy from 1946 to 1949. A majority of the electorate voted for members of Congress and a new administration that would initiate and advance health equity-focused reforms.

Truman was never successful in realizing comprehensive health reform, but he did manage to convince Congress, with the help of external advocates, to develop and pass piecemeal legislation that tackled a variety of health policy issues, including enactment of the Hill-Burton Act, which prohibited health care discrimination and provided funding to address aging health care facilities. He steered the federal government to resolve a major determinant of health, access to nutritious foods, by involving the government in the school lunch business after initiating and signing the National School Lunch Act into law. This statute was prioritized once the US military highlighted the large number of young recruits who were rejected for military service because of malnutrition during World War II and lasted thirty-five years. In 1981, President Ronald Reagan effectively eliminated this program by cutting $1.46 billion from the budget for child nutrition in an effort to reduce government spending and limit the size of government. This led to greater involvement in school lunches by private commercial interests in the food industry.

In 1946, mental health problems had also reached crisis proportions in the military, and mental health advocates saw an opportunity to grab the government's attention and elevate their agenda using a national security argument instead of a moral argument.[28] Dr. Robert Felix, the Public Health Service's assistant chief of the Hospital Division and chief of the Mental Hygiene Division, worked with advocates to develop legislation focused on bolstering mental health and pressing for its passage. They secured a hearing in Congress to highlight the mental health problems facing the country. Major General Lewis B. Hershey of the army testified that 20 percent of recruits were rejected for military service owing to mental illness, and 40 percent of military personnel were discharged owing to mental health complications.

In addition, US Surgeon General Thomas Parran Jr. (who had been an architect of the Social Security Act, which was criticized for intentionally excluding agricultural and domestic workers, largely held by women and minorities) was also invited to participate in the hearing. He testified that, at the end of World War II, half of the hospital beds were filled by people diagnosed with psychosis and, as a result, policy makers had to act to address this critical issue. These were statistics that policy makers could not ignore. Later, it would be revealed that Parran had also been the architect behind the racist Tuskegee Syphilis Study. Despite his troubled record of excluding racial and ethnic minorities in policy and exacerbating racial disparities, he played an important role in getting the National Mental Health Act of 1946 enacted into law, which for the first time in US history provided a significant amount of funding for research into the causes, prevention, and treatment of mental illness. The National Mental Health Act led to the creation in 1949 of the National Institute of Mental Health (NIMH) and helped to bolster the community mental health movement, which pushed for deinstitutionalization and integration to treat patients in their communities rather than in psychiatric hospitals. Advocates and leaders at the Community Services Branch of the NIMH continued to argue that community mental health services could promote a healthy workforce, which was "so essential to national defenses" and outlined broad steps for rehabilitation.[29]

• • •

In the mid-1800s, after a major mental health reform attempt, a movement gained traction by leveraging the political levers to abolish slavery and afford civil rights and health care to African Americans and poor whites. In the mid-1900s, after another major mental health reform push in Congress, advocates fought to expand civil rights for African Americans and end discrimination in health care. During this period, advocates wrestled with how to strategically activate grassroots advocacy, exploit the electoral system, engage all branches of government, and enact public policies to tackle inequities in America. Of all of the challenges that advocates were confronting, Martin Luther King Jr. was particularly concerned with the "need for strong and aggressive leadership from the Federal Government" because, he argued, "so far only the judicial branch of our government has rendered strong leadership. The executive and legislative branches have all too often been engaged in a conspiracy of silence and apathy." As a result, he urged advocates to mobilize in a "determined effort to arouse our government out of this apathetic slumber."[30]

Civil rights advocates did just that and used various arguments, including economics and national security, to make the case for ending segregation and discrimination against blacks. In his essay, "The Rising Tide of Racial Consciousness," Dr. Martin Luther King Jr. argued, "how we deal with [discrimination] will determine our political health as a nation and our prestige as a leader of the free world." In 1961, the federal government issued a report through the US Information Agency Office of Research and Analysis acknowledging the national security concerns for continuing to exclude and discriminate against its racial and ethnic minority citizens. According to the agency report, "for generations, this racial prejudice and discrimination have been described by foreign observers as a major defect of the American People. Enemies have instigated much bitter criticism of the caste-like status of the Negro. With the recent emergence of more than a score of nations in the two great continents populated by non-whites, the denial of equal opportunity within the United States has become an important factor in our foreign relations."[31]

The political determinants of health are, arguably, best encapsulated in the presidency of Lyndon B. Johnson. Johnson demonstrated an acute sense of the dynamics of history and politics, which helped him understand the timing needed to move progressive public policies forward. Unlike Andrew Johnson, who worked to roll back Lincoln's health equity agenda after he was assassinated, Lyndon Johnson worked to continue Kennedy's health equity agenda after Kennedy was assassinated. Among the major federal laws that were signed into law during the Johnson administration was the landmark Medicare and Medicaid legislation, which increased access to health care for many vulnerable populations and effectively prohibited overt racial segregation in the health care system. However, a course correction by the political system led to the election of Richard Nixon, who used his platform to defund and undermine many of the Johnson administration's progressive policies. This was a deep setback in the quest to move the nation closer to realizing health equity.

Jimmy Carter's 1977 election was a major step forward for federal involvement in addressing mental health issues and advancing health equity. As governor of Georgia, Carter had established the Commission to Improve Services to the Mentally and Emotionally Retarded and appointed his wife, Rosalynn, to the commission. One tremendous success during his governorship was an approximately 30 percent decrease in the number of hospitalized patients in Georgia.

Mrs. Carter decided that, if her husband were elected president, she would continue to focus on mental health reform, hoping that the beneficial results of deinstitutionalization and the creation of community mental health centers in Georgia could be repeated on a national level. Soon after his election, Carter issued an executive order establishing the President's Commission on Mental Health, the first-ever commission to deal comprehensively with the mental health system. It was tasked with determining whether people with mental illness were underserved, the proper role of the federal government in addressing their concerns, the research needed, and whether a unified approach to mental health could be developed, among other issues.

The President's Commission on Mental Health produced a seminal report in 1978 that committed to making high-quality mental health care available and affordable to those who needed it in the least restrictive setting with strengthened personal and community supports. It recommended a federal program that would create new community mental health services, particularly in underserved areas, and would encourage mental health specialists to work in those areas and ensure their training and knowledge were suitable for the needs of those populations. The report urged closing large psychiatric hospitals in favor of more comprehensive and integrated care that included community-based services and small state hospitals. After receiving the report, Carter directed Secretary Patricia Roberts Harris, head of the Department of Health, Education, and Welfare, to draft model legislation that would implement the commission's recommendations.

In May 1979, exactly 125 years after Franklin Pierce vetoed mental health reform legislation, Carter sent a message to Congress along with a draft mental health systems bill that would establish "a new partnership between the federal government and the states in the planning and provision of mental health services."[32] Passage of the final bill would take almost a year and a half. Carter's bill, the Mental Health Systems Act of 1980, aimed to restructure the community mental health center program and improve services for mentally ill people. It required states to establish community mental health centers, providing inpatient, outpatient, and emergency services, as well as consultation and education. Carter signed the act into law on October 7, 1980.

Carter's Mental Health Systems Act became law one month before the 1980 presidential election, which Carter lost to Republican Ronald Reagan. Immediately after he was inaugurated, Reagan set about dismantling many of the achievements of the Carter administration. Within months of its enactment, Reagan signed into law the Omnibus Budget Reconciliation Act in the summer of 1981, which repealed or rendered most provisions of the Mental Health Systems Act moot. The act authorized instead federal block grants to the states for mental health services. The grants provided the states only 75 to 80 percent of what they would have received under the Mental Health Systems Act. Reagan effectively ended federal funding of community treatment for the mentally ill, shifting the burden to individual state governments. It was a deep setback for mental health equity.

Immediately following Reagan's election, minority health advocates again assembled and strategized how best to advance their agenda. They gained some traction after working with the Institute of Medicine[33] to publish a report in 1981 titled *Health Care in a Context of Civil Rights*, which, along with other published research on the topic, led to the federal government's more direct and coordinated efforts to address racial and ethnic health disparities. During the next two decades, advocates would realize the passage of two pieces of legislation prioritizing health disparities reduction and elimination: (1) the nation's first ten-year public health goals, which initially prioritized reducing and then eliminating health disparities, and (2) the publication of annual reports tracking health disparities in the United States. (For a thorough description and analysis of advocacy efforts during this time, please read *150 Years of ObamaCare*.)

The Fourth Attempt: The Political Backlash and Midcourse "Correction"

The United States has long grappled with advancing health equity through the political process and codifying it into public law and policy. In 1865, seventy years after the country's government first convened, US lawmakers finally succeeded in passing the first comprehensive and inclusive law aimed at tackling the determinants of health, but that effort was short-lived. In 2010, advocates managed to not only pass another comprehensive post-Reconstruction legislation package intended to address the determinants of health but also faced a similar fate as the Freedmen's Bureau once the 2016 presidential election had concluded. Beginning in 2017, the United States faced another fork in the road relative to the advancement of health equity.

From 2008 to 2017, the electorate enabled a fundamental shift in health care with the election of Obama, almost 150 years after the first major health equity legislation was passed and signed into law. A majority of voters put in place a government that would develop a comprehensive health equity-focused policy, fix the economic and financial engines of the country, and tackle racial disparities in our educational system, among other significant reforms. Once the new government convened, advocates who championed health equity took lessons from history and successfully traversed the political minefield that had long deterred prior health equity attempts.

One lesson included using not only moral arguments but also outcomes and economic arguments to bolster their claim that health inequities should be addressed and health equity advanced in any health reform proposal. Two studies published during the 2009 health reform negotiations demonstrated the cost burden of racial and ethnic health disparities in America, conservatively estimated to be $300 billion per year at the time.[34] In addition, advocates also argued that health equity aligned with the nation's security interests as had been done in 1946 when mental health equity champions used that argument to pass legislation to prioritize mental health research and the provision of food at US schools.

Fortunately for health equity advocates, a nonpartisan, nonprofit, national security organization of retired generals, admirals, and other senior military leaders published another timely report that was released by the US Department of Defense. This report cited alarming statistics: 75 percent of young people ages seventeen to twenty-four were unfit to

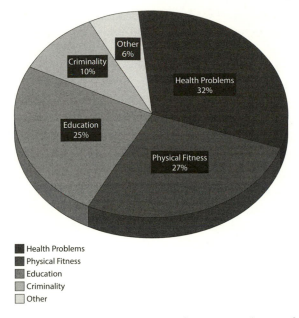

Health Problems
Physical Fitness
Education
Criminality
Other

Unfit to serve. Of all Americans between the ages of seventeen and twenty-four years old, roughly 75 percent would not qualify for military service. The top reasons are health problems, lack of physical fitness, inadequate level of education, and criminality. Mission: Readiness, *Ready, Willing, and Unable to Serve.*

serve in the US military.[35] The most common barriers for potential re-cruits were poor health, inadequate physical fitness, failure to complete high school, and a criminal record, all problems for which the political determinants played a major role in creating, perpetuating, or exacerbat-ing. According to the report:

> Nearly a third (32 percent) of all young people have health problems—other than their weight—that will keep them from serving. Many are disqualified from serving for asthma, eyesight or hearing problems, mental health issues, or recent treatment for Attention Deficit Hyperactivity Disorder. When weight problems are added in with the other health problems, over half of young adults cannot join because of health issues. Additional young people are not eligible to join because of drug or alcohol problems.[36]

A second lesson that advocates took from past attempts included the importance of timing. Past presidents had failed to gauge the opportune time to advance their health policies. Presidents Jimmy Carter, George H. W.

Bush, and Bill Clinton all suffered from long delays in getting their health bills before Congress and so lost the advantage of the honeymoon period of the earliest years of their presidencies. In contrast, President Obama pressed the need to work on his ambitious health equity agenda even before he was inaugurated as president.

According to Dr. Garth Graham, a nationally renowned health policy expert and president of the Aetna Foundation, associate clinical professor of medicine at the University of Connecticut School of Medicine, and a former deputy assistant secretary of minority health at the US Department of Health and Human Services, three of the biggest health policies, namely, the Social Security Act, Medicare and Medicaid, and the Affordable Care Act were formed in the crucible of politics. Each president and his congressional colleagues and advocates understood the politics of time: once the window of opportunity was gone it would never come back around again in their administrations. Health policy is driven by the political determinants of health in the same way. It may not be the smartest policy that gets implemented, but it may succeed because its creators recognize and successfully manipulate the politics of time.

A third lesson that advocates took from past attempts at advancing health equity included the need to persist through crisis and operate with a sense of urgency. Whereas prior presidents shelved or postponed their health reform plans when other pressing issues arose, Obama insisted on pushing ahead with his plans despite the economic crisis of 2008. It probably helped that health equity advocates were determined to achieve success this time around and kept the pressure on the president and members of Congress to finally pass a comprehensive law focused on elevating health equity. They realized that, if lost, this opportunity to enact health reform would not present itself again for decades. The urgency to get this bill passed was furthered by the notion that the Supreme Court had not demonstrated sensitivities toward past civil rights and health care issues and was chipping away protections that were included in key federal statutes.

A fourth lesson that advocates took from past attempts was uniting independent campaigns around mental health, minority health, and universal health, as well as other priorities, under one umbrella. By intentionally converging separate advocacy campaigns, health equity champions crafted a more effective, inclusive, and organic strategy, solving a problem that had challenged lawmakers for decades.[37] This evolution of a new and bolder strategy—of including all of these groups' priorities under one bill—was brilliant because everyone would have a stake in its success. In some respects, this strategy was also dangerous: it could have eventually led to the bill's demise if proponents of health equity had failed to keep the majority of interested stakeholders engaged.

A year and a half after the 2008 elections, advocates succeeded in passing and enacting the most comprehensive health equity-focused legislation in America's history. The development and passage of Obama's health law was far from static and will be explored at length in subsequent chapters. However, at this point, every successive attempt at advancing health equity allowed champions to test various approaches and develop more effective strategies for passing the agenda. Health equity champions in government and outside of government were able to avoid past mistakes or mishaps, which were necessary in laying the groundwork for the country's first comprehensive health equity policy.

No other health law has been as comprehensive as the Affordable Care Act: it extended mental health parity protections and expanded civil rights protections; required greater attention to diversity in comparative effectiveness research; ensured that critical benefits, such as maternity, behavioral health, rehabilitative, and habilitative coverage, were included as essential health benefits; authorized the largest investment in public health to tackle the most pressing chronic diseases in communities, especially those disparately impacted; promoted the integration of behavioral health and primary care; included preventive services at no cost to the consumer; and provided other opportunities for health equity-related outreach and education.

After Obama's tenure in the White House, the political pendulum started swinging back in the other direction. From a health equity perspective, the implications of the 2016 election were clear: the United States would, once again, wrestle with whether and how to advance universal health coverage, preserve civil rights, and prioritize health equity as lawmakers engaged in contentious debates over repealing and replacing the Affordable Care Act. Indeed, the 2016 election marked a critical juncture for the health law and the United States, one that would determine whether the country embraced a more accessible, equitable, and inclusive health system or reverse course toward a system of increasing health disparities. The big question was whether opponents of the Affordable Care Act would be able to follow through and successfully repeal the longest-surviving health reform law in America prioritizing health equity or whether proponents of the Affordable Care Act would stymie its repeal, unlike advocates of the Freedmen's Bureau Act?

Conclusion

In many instances, political determinants of health have played a paradoxical role in driving inequities in America—from banking, education, criminal justice, housing, employment, and health—in a system that has used the power of its platform to maintain as much of the status quo as the citizens outside would permit. Nonetheless, health equity champions have been able to amplify their message, spark a movement that highlights injustices plaguing vulnerable groups, and leverage the political determinants of health to tackle these inequities. Although few in number, they have served as lights from which many were lit. Even when that light dimmed during certain periods of our nation's history, health equity proponents continued to press forward and pushed against pseudoscience, false information, and hateful messages. They worked diligently to keep the flame of truth alive: that all individuals are created equal and are entitled to certain rights, including life, liberty, and the pursuit of happiness.

It takes resolve, patience, and drive to advance a health equity agenda in the United States because health equity is complex, and collective agreement is difficult to achieve. The history of attempts to leverage political determinants to rectify health inequities in the United States is full of frustration and discouragement. At the federal level, successes and failures in advancing health equity-focused policies and rights to resources have been realized in all branches of the government, resulting in a tug-of-war among the legislative, executive, and judicial branches. Of course, failures are more numerous than successes, but through the unwavering efforts of advocates, major victories in concretizing health rights have been realized, especially over the past fifty years, with congressional efforts leading to more universal expansion of health rights followed by administrative and judicial efforts.

Statutorily, advocates secured the right to health care for individuals sixty-five years and older and those younger than sixty-five years old who have a disability. They secured health care rights for those who fall below the federal poverty level and for uninsured children from low-income families. Advocates also statutorily secured the right to be screened and stabilized at hospital emergency departments, the right to parity in coverage for mental health benefits and medical/surgical benefits, and a right to access health insurance coverage and protections for those with preexisting conditions. These were incremental, but significant, reforms in the quest to increase access and prioritize health equity.

Judicially, advocates secured limited rights, including the right to privacy, the right to use contraception, the right to make reproductive decisions, the right to decide to have an abortion, the right to health care for prisoners, and the right to refuse treatment. However, the Supreme Court has held that there is no right to government funding for most of these limited, judicially secured rights, leaving the decision to Congress about whether to fund such access. The Supreme Court has also limited statutorily gained rights, such as protections under the Americans with Disabilities Act and the Mental Health Parity Act, but it has never found a health law unconstitutional.

When the Supreme Court has wrestled with whether to expand additional rights and failed to do so, Congress has statutorily expanded those rights. In *Youngberg v. Romeo*, 457 US 307 (1982), the Supreme Court was confused about whether and how to extend a right for habilitation[38] coverage, but during negotiations involving the Affordable Care Act, policy makers, almost three decades later, included provisions deeming habilitation coverage an essential benefit because research had by then shown how favorable it was to overall health.

Our current understanding of health disparities demonstrates that not one factor but multiple interacting determinants drive inequities in health care, in large part because of our political system. As Professor Johan P. Mackenbach of Erasmus University in Rotterdam reminds us, "engage in research identifying causal effects of political variables (structures, processes, outputs) on population health" because "most of the effects of politics on population health are likely to be less immediately visible in routinely collected data."[39] Unless we engage in this interdisciplinary research and demonstrate the causal link between political determinants and health inequities, we will lose ground in the argument that health inequities today are primarily the result of social factors, not political factors, which will leave us with no legal or political remedy to leverage.

Very few public policies, programs, initiatives, and laws employ an equity lens, which is problematic given the United States' stated goal of becoming a more healthy and equitable society.[40] Rather than despair, advocates have an opportunity to address not only the negative outcomes of health disparities but also the imbalance of inputs in the political process. Addressing this complex issue is even more critical today considering that in the near future many of the populations that tend to experience significant disparities in health status and care are expected to comprise a majority of America's population. The problem will only become more pronounced with the rising incidence of obesity and chronic diseases, illnesses and disorders fueled in part by policies allowing the infusion of obesity-causing ingredients in our diets, government support for polluting industries that continue to contribute to climate change, and an increasingly vulnerable aging population.

It is incumbent on health equity proponents to work diligently to ensure that policy makers recognize the shortsightedness of taking a reactionary approach to health policies—which has been the nation's response during our history to direct threat, outbreak, or other national security reasons—and instead take a proactive approach to eliminate health inequities. This can be done by understanding and addressing political determinants of health. Chapter 3 outlines a detailed model of these political determinants to assist community members, researchers, scholars, leaders, and policy makers as they continue to advance health equity.

3

The Political Determinants of Health Model

The idea of a Constitution that is still being perfected but is ever more inclusive is something that will drive me.—*Ruth Bader Ginsburg, US Supreme Court Justice*

In many respects, our health system continues to grow more intricate as it tries to move away from a patchwork of fragmented components to a system that pushes and pulls providers and consumers toward better health outcomes and value in a complex ecosystem. Underlying this complexity and stifling its resiliency is a major issue that has eluded researchers, scientists, health care leaders, and policy makers for decades—health inequities. As our attention has been focused on addressing health inequities downstream at the individual level, one person at a time, and midstream at the community level, less attention has been focused upstream on a broader level to address the structures, processes, and outputs that result in the inequities we have today. Until we can recognize their impact and develop community-centric, evidence-based, and effective upstream solutions to tackle the factors that cause and intensify these inequities, we will make little progress in improving the American health care system.

In the United States, as in all countries of the world, the nation's health is not an organic outcome. It is not a coincidence that certain groups of Americans experience higher premature death rates than others. It is not a fluke that some groups experience poverty for generations, blocked from attaining the American dream. Sometimes we do not see the depths of the problem, until we start digging and examining their root causes and distribution, and then it becomes apparent that one major factor has exacerbated the disparities in health status: our political system. This system has not always valued each group equally or realized the long-term implications of policies on the health of its citizenry. High obesity rates, maternal mortality, infant mortality, gun violence, depression, opioid addiction, substance use disorders, diabetes, heart disease, cancer, HIV/AIDS, and many other health problems can be firmly linked to political action or inaction.

Today, we recognize that a variety of forces collectively impact our health and determine our life expectancy, including social, environmental, economic, behavioral health, health care, and genetic factors.[1] Too often we stop at those drivers of inequities, failing to dig even further to understand the bigger picture. As a result, we miss the link between these generally accepted determinants of health and the political determinants of health. These political determinants of health inequitably distribute social, medical, and other determinants and create structural barriers to equity for population groups that lack power and privilege.

For different reasons, we tend to shy away from the role that political forces have played in creating, maintaining, and increasing the inequities we observe today and the impact they have on all the forces that affect our health. We also fail to recognize how past political determinants have been leveraged to advance policies to bolster health equity. Joseph P. Kennedy, a former ambassador and father of President John F. Kennedy, understood that political outcomes were not accidental. He stated in 1960, "There are no accidents in politics."[2] Our political system engages in a predictable pattern relative to the advancement of health equity. If that is true, then it is absolutely important that health equity proponents understand the history, the politics, the policies, and the tools that have been and can be used to advance their agenda. This chapter is intended to introduce a new model to examine the single greatest determinant in producing and perpetuating health inequities in the United States and the interventions available to elevate health equity: the political determinants of health.

Like many industrialized nations, the United States focuses its resources primarily on increasing access to health services and improving the quality of care provided to consumers. And while the US life expectancy rate has increased by approximately thirty years over the past century, only five of those years can be attributed to health care, according to an Institute of Medicine report.[3] A study by Drs. Margarita Alegría, Debra Joy Pérez, and Sandra Williams in *Health Affairs* found that "the impact of medical care, socioeconomic, lifestyle, and environmental factors on the health production function of the U.S. population show that additional medical care use is limited in increasing life expectancy."[4] Although it is true that health care plays a critical role in overall health status and life expectancy, we should not solely focus on health care at the expense of

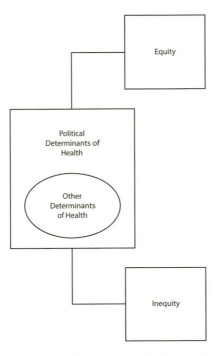

The relationship between the political determinants of health and the other determinants of health.

social, economic, behavioral health, and environmental determinants. Since these determinants of health operate simultaneously and collectively to impact us, we should be focused on addressing them in tandem.

Over the years, as our knowledge has increased, several frameworks have been developed to explore how various determinants of health, including health care, environmental, and social factors, create or contribute to health inequities. Some scholars have assigned a relative percentage of impact of each determinant on overall health status: health care has been assigned an approximate impact of 10-20 percent; environmental determinants, such as toxic waste sites, natural disasters, or climate change have been assigned a 20 percent impact; and social determinants, such as education, housing, transportation, and employment, among others, have been assigned a 20-40 percent impact.[5] When these and other factors are mismanaged, including genetics and behavioral health, they lead to racial, disability, sex, gender, income, and geographic disparities among particular communities.

Furthermore, when differences in health status are significantly associated with social disadvantages, researchers have labeled the differences as health inequities. According to a landmark study conducted by the World Health Organization, these health inequities, in most cases, are systematic and avoidable, facilitated and exacerbated by circumstances in which people live, work, pray, play, and contend with illness, intensified by social, economic, and political influences at global, national, and local levels.[6] So, why should this matter to our policy makers and leaders? Because health inequities, if left unchecked, undermine a country's full potential. They reduce its productivity, impair its economic growth, and weaken its national security.

In recognition of the social determinants of health's outsized impact on our life expectancy and health status, Professor Sir Michael Marmot and other notable researchers in recent years have increasingly focused attention on examining these generally broad determinants of health, "the conditions in which people are born, grow, work, live, and age, and the *wider set of forces and systems shaping* the conditions of daily life."[7] These social variables, it is argued, determine whether we have access to safe and quality housing, education, employment, transportation, and grocery stores that sell healthy food options. They result in a cycle of poor nutrition, poor health, and poor performance in school or at work and increased crime rates, health costs, and poverty.

It is often difficult to differentiate whether health inequities originate from political factors or whether the political factors are masked by social factors or other determinants. This chapter will discuss the greatest instigator among the "wider set of forces and systems"—the political determinants of health—focusing on its role in creating, exacerbating, or removing systemic barriers and prioritizing health equity. It will argue that we must continue to move even further upstream, understanding the interconnection between all of the determinants of health and the overarching influence that political determinants have had on all of the determinants.[8] It will also discuss how these political determinants have been the main drivers for the state of health and the alarming inequities in health that we experience in the United States and in other countries.

Political determinants of health involve the systematic process of structuring relationships, distributing resources, and administering power, operating simultaneously in ways that mutually reinforce or influence one another to shape opportunities that either advance health equity or exacerbate health inequities. This new model, which focuses on three major aspects of the political determinants—voting, government, and policy—will provide another lens through which to examine the structures,[9] processes,[10] and outputs[11] that enable inequities to systematically develop and flourish. It provides a multidisciplinary framework to address the multiple, complex factors affecting the entire life continuum, which are responsible for hastening premature death for some and extending life for others.[12]

Admittedly, the political determinants of health are more charged and less palatable than other determinants, such as those in the social sphere. Yet, we ignore them at our peril, for they disproportionately influence and impact all the determinants of health. They exacerbate health inequities, including early death and disability, and contribute to poor health outcomes experienced by low-income individuals, rural and frontier communities, racial and ethnic communities, sexual and gender minorities, people with disabilities, people with mental illnesses and substance use disorders, military veterans, and others experiencing systemic barriers to health-enhancing opportunities.[13] Overall, health inequities in the United States can be traced back to a political determinant even when the inequities are deemed to result from an environmental, social, economic, health care, or behavioral health determinant. The political determinants are the instigators of the causes. They are the determinants of the determinants.

One example includes the refusal to establish and expand Medicaid after the passage of the Medicare and Medicaid Act in 1965 and after passage of the Affordable Care Act in 2010, which occurred primarily in southern states, the area of the country that experiences the highest cost and mortality burden owing to health inequities. Another example includes the National Rifle Association's effective lobbying to push lawmakers to terminate funding for gun violence research at the Centers for Disease Control and Prevention. This congressional amendment was added to a larger funding bill via a policy rider known as the Dickey Amendment, which the federal government passed in 1996. The ban on funding for gun violence research at the CDC resulted in a dearth of research involving the impact of firearms on a community's health, and has resulted in additional state laws being enacted such as the physician gag laws preventing doctors, especially pediatricians, from discussing whether there is a gun in the home. And outside of the United States, in England, after the government changed their salt policy in 2011 to allow the food industry greater flexibility to set and monitor targets for curbing salt intake, more Britons developed gastric cancer and heart disease than would have happened under the older strict governmental policy.[14]

However, although the political determinants have created and sustained inequities in health, opportunities exist to intervene in the political process to overcome these avoidable and remediable problems and to advance health equity in all communities. Research shows that targeted policy approaches have measurably improved the health of many Americans and that health equity is possible through policy action.[15] Health policies that focused on eliminating disparities and employing culturally tailored approaches, including childhood immunizations, breast cancer prevention and treatment, tobacco control, health enterprise zones, and maternal and child health, demonstrate this fact. Moreover, other types of public policies have been shown to increase health equity, including those that have increased the minimum wage. According to research, "a dollar increase in the minimum wage above the federal law was associated with 1% to 2% decrease in low birth weight births and a 4% decrease in postneonatal mortality."[16] This one-dollar increase in the minimum wage across all states would have led to "2790 fewer low birth weight births and 518 fewer postneonatal deaths" in one year.[17]

Health, wealth, educational, and income inequities are all intrinsically and inextricably linked. They persist owing to political determinants, including *legalized* discrimination in housing, education, transportation, employment, and exclusionary city zoning laws.[18] Too often, disconnected and undervoiced communities are disproportionately burdened with overcoming these inequities and negative outcomes and therefore cannot confront the disjointed political systems and institutions that created, fueled, and continued them. These systems develop or enforce policy actions or inactions orchestrated by a complex web of local to international agents. At each stage of the political process, advocates, engaged in creating and expanding a health equity-focused program for underresourced populations, need to be aware of vulnerabilities. They may find themselves challenged by opponents who relentlessly look for opportunities to snip individual threads in the safety net to unravel it legislatively, administratively, or judicially.

In some respects, health equity can be likened to a rope where the political determinants of health collectively are the forces that twist and tighten each strand, which represent the other determinants of health. The political determinants of health have made it difficult, but not impossible, to later disentangle the other determinants of health or loosen the strands to thoughtfully address the drivers of health inequities. This force can work to the benefit or detriment of health equity, depending on consumer, government, or corporate stakeholder interest. There is a balancing act between the three, but corporate interests rule unless the policy significantly hurts consumer or government interests.

The Political Determinants of Health Explained

To tackle the broad and collateral effects of the political determinants of health, we can target the three major aspects that interact in various ways to advance or hinder health equity: voting, government, and policy. The first political determinant of health, *voting*, puts in place or allows you to bypass the decision makers, the people charged with creating or executing policy that affects everyone, regardless of whether you have engaged in the political process. However, only electing individuals aligned with your position does not guarantee that health equity will be prioritized, since the policy maker will join a system of competing interests where policy savvy and political acumen are critical. The second political determinant of health, *government*, provides a mechanism for decision makers to keep, enforce, or change the status quo by reinforcing existing policy, doing away with existing policy, or creating new policy at the local, state, regional, and federal levels. The third political determinant of health, *policy*, essentially concretizes or codifies the final decision or action. Those three aspects of the political determinants of health are affected by carefully planned and executed advocacy efforts, which is at the heart of this whole process.

Although this notion may come as a surprise for some health equity advocates, two competing interests must align to effect changes leveraging the political determinants of health—human interests and commercial interests. As is the case with most advocacy efforts in the United States, the likelihood of their success depends on how palatable they are to commercial interests and whether there is an investment value to the government.[19] This fact is even more pronounced when you consider that over the past twenty years, the US Chamber of Commerce, which is the "world's largest business organization representing the interests of more than 3 million businesses of all sizes, sectors, and regions,"[20] has played a major role in election and lobbying activities, consistently ranking as the top spender on these activities.[21]

In 1999, the chamber spent approximately $18.6 million, which progressively increased to a staggering $144 million at the beginning of the Obama administration once health reform negotiations started. Every election year, the Chamber of Commerce substantially increased its spending from the year before. Spending on health care lobbying by the chamber and other health care trade groups has "consistently outpaced other sector-related lobbying year after year," with a staggering $555 million spent on health care lobbying in 2017.[22] As a result, it is unsurprising that rarely does an advocacy initiative succeed if it significantly interferes with or undermines commercial activities or national security. Therefore, it is important that you understand the deeply rooted interplay between the commercial interests and the political determinants of health.[23]

Here are some examples of times when the political system intervened to address a serious health policy issue once it aligned with a commercial interest and there was an investment value to the government. Consider, for example, the 1798 law providing health care to sailors to prevent infections and thus protect trade. Or the provision of health care to members of the military to ensure they are fit to serve and defend the nation in times of war. Initially, the government's investment value centered on protecting its military and trade systems from the spread of infectious diseases which were the leading causes of death in America for most of its history.[24] Today, noninfectious diseases are the leading causes of death, which is disquieting in light of a recent study showing "that obesity is the leading medical disqualifier that prevents otherwise qualified Americans from joining the military."[25]

After mental health advocates unsuccessfully tried to pass mental health reforms in the mid-1800s, almost one hundred years later, they successfully advocated for mental health legislation to establish a national institute to study mental illness in 1946. They achieved this by strategically developing arguments that highlighted how the bill was necessary to prevent a national security crisis among young people who were increasingly becoming more unfit for military service. Fifty years later, after the passage of national legislation to study mental illness, advocates, once again, were able to tie how their efforts to bolster legal protections against discrimination in mental health benefits aligned with commercial interests and an investment value to the government by arguing it would keep employees productive in the workforce and thus add to the country's economic output.

Other examples involve the provision of nutritious school lunches beginning in 1946 after World War II to combat malnutrition among children and youth as well as the provision of health insurance coverage to all children whose household income falls under a certain level to enable them to receive the health services they need. The investment value to the government in providing food and health care was to ensure that these young people would stand a better chance of becoming productive citizens and fit to serve in the military. In some cases, the commercial interest and government's investment value were more sinister, such as when it provided inoculations to Native Americans "against smallpox to make it safer for the military to dispossess them"[26] or when it provided inoculations to Chinese residents in San Francisco to prevent the spread of the bubonic plague. Advocates who have understood this notion of demonstrating how their advocacy issue aligns with commercial interests and a government investment value have been more successful in advancing their health policy agendas, such as Medicare and Medicaid, the Americans with Disabilities Act, the Mental Health Parity and Addiction Equity Act, and the Patient Protection and Affordable Care Act.

The illustration on this page depicts the political determinants of health model. Its interconnecting, or circular, arrows show that the political determinants of health operate simultaneously in ways that mutually

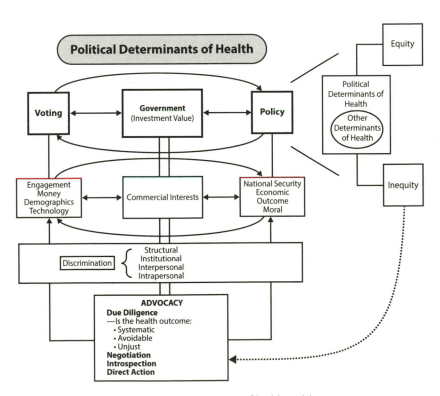

The political determinants of health model.

reinforce one another and concurrently impact or are impacted by a continuum of interacting barriers and interventions. Advocates must overcome these barriers and leverage interventions to advance health equity-focused policies and address other competing and equally complex determinants of health. The bracket refers to the relationship between the political determinants of health and all the other determinants of health, which collectively affect the creation and advancement of health equity. This is a continual strategic process that does not end once a policy is realized but requires constant monitoring by advocates to determine whether a policy or governmental action is positively or negatively affecting the determinants of health and advancing equity. The sections that follow break down each section of the political determinants of health model.

The First Political Determinant of Health: Voting

In the United States, voting is a fundamental civic duty, yet many individuals fail to recognize or take for granted voting's impact on their health, well-being, and life expectancy. Despite evidence that shows the individual health benefits from voting, the less healthy individuals are, the less likely they are to vote and the less likely they are to have their

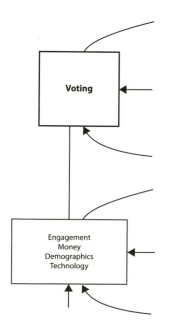

Voting as a political determinant of health.

concerns meaningfully addressed. Studies have shown a correlation between voting behaviors and a broad index of poor health.[27] Voting is arguably the most important aspect of the political determinants because it not only affords us an opportunity to directly engage in and work on immediate policy solutions to the issues affecting our communities but also installs the policy makers who will form the decisions and drive our agenda on a macro level. Moreover, voting provides an opportunity to address the long-term biological and societal consequences of the determinants of health and enables the decisions, research, programs, and policies that allow us to tackle these issues. Despite this information, many apathetic individuals do not engage in electoral politics because they do not believe government works for them.[28] Voter apathy has been steadily rising since 2004, according to the US Census Bureau, and is now the second leading reason cited for not voting in the United States. Given the connection between voting and health opportunities, advocates must work to overcome these challenges.

related to trust and transparency

According to the Pew Research Center, the United States trails most developed countries in voter turnout, ranking twenty-six out of thirty-two countries, with 55.7 percent of the voting-age population turning out to vote in 2016.[29] Both of the United States' neighbors, Canada and Mexico, outrank it along with Australia, Israel, Greece, Czech Republic, Slovakia, South Korea, and the United Kingdom. Out of 245.5 million individuals in the United States who were eighteen and older in 2016, approximately 157.6 million reported being registered to vote, and only about 136.8 million cast a vote in the presidential election.[30] The percentage of voters who cast a vote in any given election usually ranges in the fifties, "from just under 50% in 1996, when Bill Clinton was re-elected, to just over 58% in 2008, when Barack Obama won the White House."[31] When disaggregated by race or ethnicity, voter turnout is significantly lower among racial and ethnic groups, including African Americans, Asian Americans, and Hispanic and Native Americans. However, despite the disparities in voter turnout among certain racial and ethnic groups overall, with the exception of Asian Americans, there has been an increase in voter participation rates for all racial groups from 1996 onward until the 2016 elections when the African American voter turnout rate dropped significantly and Hispanic voter turnout dipped slightly. According to the Census Bureau, while there was a spike in the number of registered voters who did not vote owing to their dislike of the candidates or did not think their votes would matter in 2016, more than one in ten Americans who were registered to vote and did not vote

related to access

combo of trust and access

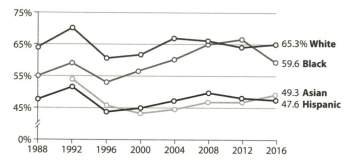

Eligible US voters who say they voted, by race (in percentages). J. M. Krogstad and M. H. Lopez, "Black Voter Turnout Fell in 2016, Even as a Record Number of Americans Cast Ballots," Pew Research Center, May 12, 2017, https://www.pewresearch.org/fact-tank/2017/05/12/black-voter-turnout-fell-in-2016-even-as-a-record-number-of-americans-cast-ballots/.

cited illness or disability as the reason.[32] Since 2000, disability or illness has been one of the top reasons given for disengagement from the political process, which is problematic given how important electoral engagement is to shaping policies upstream that ultimately impact virtually everyone living within the country.

Art Collins, chairman of the board of trustees at Morehouse School of Medicine and an expert on the political process, has stated, "there are four factors, which are not usually discussed in tandem, that define our current state of national political affairs and policy development. When considered together they explain our governing dysfunction and mistrust by the public."[33] These four factors can be categorized generally as (1) engagement, (2) money, (3) demographics, and (4) technology. To effectively address the political determinants of health, advocates must overcome and, in turn, leverage these factors.

Engagement

The first factor is overt exclusion from civic *engagement* through historical methods of gerrymandering which includes coercive attempts to restrict ballot access of citizens on the downside of elite American privilege. Opportunities for civic engagement, have been stymied by continual efforts to restrict or suppress voting by groups who have limited power and privilege, including the parochial nature of congressional redistricting and the process by which we choose our representatives. Voting restrictions, such as voter identification laws, purging voter rolls of irregular voters, minimizing the opportunities for early voting, requiring proof of citizenship, and closing or moving polling places farther away from voters, have disproportionately affected racial and ethnic minority communities and lower-socioeconomic status individuals. After the 2018 midterm elections, several Republican-controlled state legislatures increased efforts "to change voting-related rules in ways that might reduce future voter turnout" in competitive states owing to demographic and political trends.[34]

After Democrats flipped two congressional and twelve legislative seats and came close to winning a US Senate seat, Texas state lawmakers considered adding criminal penalties for people who improperly fill out voter registration forms, which would have made the legislation one of the strictest voter suppression laws in the United States. In Arizona, after Republicans lost control of all statewide offices when Democrats won four of the nine seats and a US Senate seat, state lawmakers proposed new voting rules that could make it more complicated to cast an early ballot. In Tennessee, after increased voter registrations in Nashville and Memphis, which have been Democratic strongholds, Republican lawmakers proposed penalizing groups involved in voter registration drives that submit incomplete forms. Proponents of these proposed policy efforts argue that they "are needed to maintain the integrity of voter rolls and prevent fraud."[35] However, opponents "argue that the policies are designed to dampen turnout among younger, nonwhite and poorer voters, who are less likely to back Republicans," especially in increasingly racially diverse states such as Texas and Arizona.[36]

Voting rights are essential for creating and advancing health equity. When voter suppression occurs, people most impacted by inequities and who need a fair adjudication of their issues are the same people who are actively locked out of the political system. These voter restrictions usually follow another important, but often ignored, tactic used for political gain, redistricting, which has been increasingly employed over the past twenty years.[37] Redistricting plays a significant role in disenfranchising racial and ethnic groups. Every ten years, states engage in redrawing their state legislative district and congressional lines after the census. Redistricting is a chief instigator in preventing the integration of diverse perspectives across the political continuum by segregating and concentrating racial and ethnic groups in as few districts as possible. It has resulted in elected policy makers not having to address particular issues raised by minority groups.

Recently, attention has focused on protecting the redistricting process from abuse. According to the Brennan Center for Justice, "while the vast majority of jurisdictions continue to use their state legislatures for drawing districts, there is a growing movement toward alternative approaches to map drawing. Citizen-driven ballot initiatives sparked redistricting reform in Arizona in 2000 and in California in 2008 and 2010. Since then, Colorado, Michigan, Missouri, New York, Ohio, and Utah have also adopted various types of reforms."[38] As sometimes happens when the majority party in government is unhappy with the passage of a citizen-driven ballot initiative that threatens their status quo, the Missouri House of Representatives passed a proposal just five months after the 2018 midterm elections, which they will offer to the voters in the next election. This legislatively driven proposal is intended to undo a voter-approved constitutional amendment titled, "Clean Missouri," which would appoint a nonpartisan demographer to draft state House and Senate maps after the 2020 Census.[39] The Missouri legislature decided it would be more fair and competitive not to have a nonpartisan demographer conduct the redistricting process but to have bipartisan panels to redraw districts, as was done previously. Advocates should inform themselves of how these voting restrictions have been used in the past to disenfranchise groups and continue to connect the dots about how these efforts impact the health of communities.

Money

The second factor that has impacted our current political state and policy development includes the unlimited nature, manipulation, and concealment of *money* in campaign finance and lobbying and, more importantly, the negative use of such funding, including the constant stream of media funding by groups invested in maintaining the status quo. Campaign financing has increased significantly from 1998 to 2016. For congressional elections, the cost went from a little over $1.6 billion to a little over $4.1 billion.[40] During that same period, the cost of presidential elections went from approximately $1.4 billion to almost $2.4 billion. Collectively, the 2016 presidential and congressional elections cost a whopping $6.5 billion.

The amount of money spent per candidate to participate in US elections versus other similarly situated countries is astounding. Consider, for example, that, in the United States, candidates for the House of Representatives spent approximately $500,000 and candidates for the Senate spent approximately $1.5 million in 2016. In contrast, candidates for par-

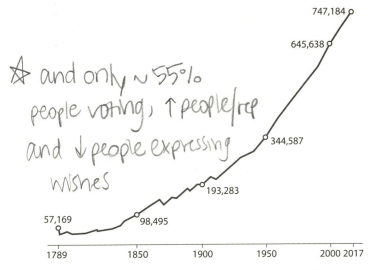

747,184

645,638

☆ and only ~55% people voting, ↑ people/rep and ↓ people expressing wishes

344,587

193,283

57,169

98,495

1789   1850   1900   1950   2000 2017

The number of people represented by one US House member. "U.S. Population Keeps Growing, but House of Representatives Is Same Size as in Taft Era," Pew Research Center, May 31, 2018, https://www.pewresearch.org/fact-tank/2018/05/31/u-s-population-keeps-growing-but-house -of-representatives-is-same-size-as-in-taft-era/.

liament in Canada spent between $12,000 and $90,000, which mirrors other countries.

Lobbying expenditures in the United States went from $1.45 billion in 1998 to a staggering $3.51 billion in 2010 at the height of the Affordable Care Act negotiations before leveling off on average to a little over $3 billion thereafter. As a result, advocates can expect to see significant spending on advocacy activities, depending on the health policy issue and its implications on health care payment. Consider, for example, that opponents of an advocacy effort outspent proponents five to one in the case of a citizen-initiated ballot measure, such as Colorado's universal health care initiative, or fifteen to one in the case of the Affordable Care Act.

Demographics

The third factor that affects our current political affairs and policy development includes *demographic* changes and the growing physical disconnect between those represented and those who represent them. "When was the last time you saw or spoke to your member of Congress?" In the US House of Representatives, there is one House member for every

747,000 Americans, up from one House member for every 209,447 people in 1910. In 2017, there was one representative for every 747,184 people, making it the highest population-to-representative ratio among peer countries for the thirty-five nations in the Organisation for Economic Co-operation and Development. This is the highest it has ever been in the United States, which has increased disconnect between politicians and their constituency. This disconnect between representatives and their constituents is expected to increase as the population grows to over four hundred million by 2058.

Compounding this disconnection is changing demographics. The US population continues to grow, and it is expected that, collectively, racial and ethnic minorities will be the leading population group in the United States in twenty-five years. Since 2011, diversity has increased with each successive Congress but an increase in the passage of bills that advance health equity has not occurred. In Congress, as in most legislatures across the United States, leaders who have initiated and advanced these health equity-focused bills have usually come from communities most impacted by inequities.

At the beginning of 2017, racial and ethnic minorities made up approximately 38 percent of the US population, but in the 115th Congress,

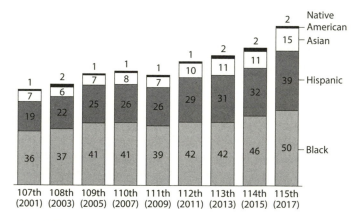

Racial and ethnic diversity trends in the US Congress. "For the Fifth Time in a Row, the New Congress Is the Most Racially and Ethnically Diverse Ever," Pew Research Center, February 8, 2019, https://www.pewresearch.org/fact-tank/2019/02/08/for-the-fifth-time-in-a-row-the-new-congress-is-the-most-racially-and-ethnically-diverse-ever/.

nonwhites (including African Americans, Hispanics, Asian-Pacific Islanders, and Native Americans) represented nearly 19 percent of the members. At the beginning of the 116th Congress in January 2019, nonwhites represented 21 percent of the members. While nonwhites have made some significant headway in getting elected to the House of Representatives, it continues to be difficult for them to secure Senate or gubernatorial seats. It is still difficult to draw the attention of the House to address health inequities. This demographic shift will require the United States, for economic and national security interests, to be more intentionally inclusive in its political system and in elevating health equity priorities.

Technology

The fourth factor affecting current political state and policy development is the impact of *technology* as it permeates and exacerbates the issues previously discussed. Since the turn of the twenty-first century, the use of technology to engage and influence the electorate has proliferated. From big data and data analytics to understand what is effective in a campaign to social media such as Twitter, Facebook, Instagram, and LinkedIn to share information or spread misinformation, technology will continue to be a major force in elections, helping to limit or advance civic education and engagement as we work to remedy our current state of affairs and more effectively address the political determinants of health.

The interventions or strategies employed at the front end of the political process—voting—provide the first tools that can be used either to elevate or to undermine efforts to overcome the barriers preventing the enfranchisement of certain groups, and they can also be used directly to advance health equity-focused policies. Voting not only provides an opportunity to elect policy makers who are charged with governing, initiating, or keeping policies but also provides an opportunity for individuals, unions, or corporations to initiate ballot measures, effectively bypassing policy makers. Through these ballot measures, you enact or quash policies that these legislators may have been afraid or unwilling to pass or implement or may have passed without respect to the opposition against the measure.

Ballot Augmentation

According to the National Conference of State Legislatures, twenty-four states allow citizens to bypass their state legislature by initiating proposed statutes and constitutional amendments on the ballot, and all states permit citizens to vote on ballot measures in one form or another, through popular and legislative referenda.[41] Recent health equity–related, citizen-initiated, and passed ballot measures include the restoration of voting rights for felons by constitutional amendment in Florida; the passage of Medicaid expansion statutes in Maine, Nebraska, Idaho, and Utah; and the passage of paid sick leave in Massachusetts.

Since 1871, when Minnesota initiated the first health care ballot measure, approximately 325 health care ballot measures have been successfully initiated and passed in states across the United States. Between 2008 and 2018, approximately 214 health care ballot measures were initiated, but only 55 were successfully passed across the United States.[42] The other 159 measures did not even make the ballot.[43] This may be owing to the tremendous time, money, resources, and effort involved in initiating ballot measures, but with an approximately 25 percent success rate, it is nonetheless a credible, but underutilized option to advance or impede health equity, especially since no ballot measure that explicitly focuses on health equity has ever been introduced or passed.

Advocates choosing ballot augmentation should be aware of potential impediments before engaging in this enormous undertaking. Some ballots may be rejected because not enough signatures were collected as required or opponents may initiate lawsuits and attack advertisements challenging the measure. Other advocates may have missed the deadline for filing the measure. Sometimes advocates decide not to focus resources on states where the ballot may fail and focus, instead, on other states where passage seems more likely. Sometimes an initiated and certified ballot measure is removed after mutual agreement by competing groups, such as unions or corporations, or it may be withdrawn due to federal health policy circumstances. In other instances, the secretary of state may deem it unqualified, resulting in "indeterminable state or local government costs depending on how it is interpreted and applied by the courts."[44] Moreover, sometimes it can be approved for circulation by a secretary of state, rejected as a violation of a state law, and then overturned by a court and still not reach the ballot because of failure to collect the required signatures. Advocates should remember all the available tools to elevate their agenda, including the rarely and seemingly elusive ballot augmentation.

The Second Political Determinant of Health: Government and the Structural, Institutional, Interpersonal, and Intrapersonal Barriers

While we work to eliminate voter apathy, prevent voter disenfranchisement, and build awareness of the connection between voting and health, advocates should also educate, reeducate, and reconnect individuals to their governments at all levels and measurably reaffirm that government action truly affects the lives of everyone. Voting, by itself, without continued engagement in the political process, will not suffice to meaningfully address inequities. Justice Sandra Day O'Connor, the first female justice appointed to the US Supreme Court, echoed this sentiment, declaring "you have citizens who don't understand how government works and they're kind of soured on it. All they do is criticize. They have no idea that they can make things happen. As a citizen, you need to know how to be a part of it, how to express yourself—and not just by voting."[45]

For the second political determinant of health—government—advocates must overcome or leverage the simultaneous and mutually reinforcing

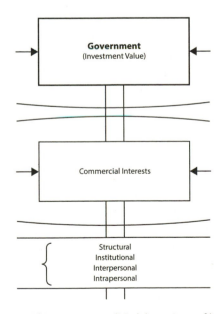

Governmental and commercial interests as a political determinant of health and their intersection with structural, institutional, interpersonal, and intrapersonal barriers.

levels of the social-ecological model[46] and structural barriers. This includes understanding the interplay between intrapersonal, interpersonal, institutional, and structural barriers sanctioned by government through the introduction or nonintroduction, the enactment or nonenactment, the enforcement or nonenforcement, or the claw back or repeal of policy. These factors or barriers cut across not only all government components but also all the political determinants of health and are responsible for the dearth of inclusive and equitable policies. Even the judicial branch, which prides itself on being an objective, nonpolitical branch of government, is not immune from political pressure because "political realities, as always, put a constraint on judicial reasoning."[47] The Supreme Court seems to have had a moment of clarity on this point when it suggested that the Constitution can evolve with changing public attitudes, stating "times can blind us to certain truths, and later generations can see that laws once thought necessary and proper, in fact, serve only to oppress."[48]

In the United States, history has shown us that when one or two branches of government have elevated rights or protections for a minority group another branch usually swoops in to limit or retract those rights once it appears that the protected group is on the brink of attaining power. Sometimes, after time has passed, the very branches that orchestrated the effort to bolster protections and rights for a minority group may end up terminating them. These structural, institutional, interpersonal, and intrapersonal barriers make it difficult, but not impossible, to broaden the inclusivity of policies and other political initiatives. To get to equity, one must conduct the necessary research or collect the existing evidence to demonstrate the fallacy of arguments raised to justify these barriers and understand the historical context and the legal and political system in order to maneuver around these barriers.

The majority of policy makers in the United States, whether federal, state, or local, made it to the government by way of institutions and professions[49] that are out of reach for most Americans. They tend to be more educated[50] and affluent than the people they represent, and they tend to focus on informing, developing, or executing policies that govern their professional backgrounds and experiences. While it may be easier to secure an elected office at the local or state levels without any past political experience, once a person runs for federal office, it becomes rare for them to successfully gain the position without past political experience, which adds another layer of difficulty for those who come from backgrounds (usually those who experience inequities) that diverge from these prevalent characteristics of most policy makers. Consequently, although there has been an increase in diversity in the halls of power, whether legislatively, administratively, or judicially, few policies have been developed and enacted focusing on health equity.

Discrimination is institutionalized in the very fabric of our society. Therefore, unsurprisingly, our governments, organizations, and associations are doubly infected with the same social maladies of racism, misogyny, ableism, and homophobia as the people in our society that operate within them. Unsurprisingly, our governments, organizations, and associations mirror as many of the biases as the people in our society who operate within them. According to the National Academies of Sciences, "organizational rules sometime evolve out of past histories (including past histories of racism) that are not easily reconstructed, and such rules may appear quite neutral on the surface." If these embedded processes result in differential treatment or produce differential outcomes, then the results may be unjustifiably discriminatory and hence are referred to as structural discrimination.[51] Dr. Camara P. Jones, a past president of the American Public Health Association and a leading expert on racism, has stated that this form of discrimination manifests itself both in access to material conditions such as quality housing, education, and health services as well as access to power such as disparate access to information, resources, and voice.[52] And according to Dr. David R. Williams, a professor of public health at the Harvard T.H. Chan School of Public Health and a leading expert on the impact of discrimination, there is a link between discrimination, as manifested both in access to material conditions and power, and poor health among minority groups.[53]

The Supreme Court, which has final authority regarding the US Constitution, has acknowledged ongoing structural and institutional discrimination and explicitly stated, "vestiges of past segregation by state decree do remain in our society and in our schools. Past wrongs to the black race, wrongs committed by the state and in its name, are a stubborn fact of history. And stubborn facts of history linger and persist. But though we cannot escape our history, *neither must we overstate its consequences in fixing legal responsibilities.*"[54] This declaration from the highest Court in the land is alarming for several reasons.

First, the Supreme Court fails to take into account the evidence from a broad spectrum of research in public health, medicine, science, nursing, allied health, economics, sociology, psychology, and social work, demonstrating the impact that these vestiges of slavery, segregation, and subsequent unjustified discrimination have on population groups. These studies show that there is accelerated aging among groups, or as Professor Arline T. Geronimus at the University of Michigan School of Public Health has concluded, biological weathering to the constant adversity. The impact of racism, homophobia, and sexism has long-lasting and severe consequences. Epigenetic and psychological research shows how trauma has affected generations of Native Americans, African Americans, Latinx, and other groups and shows how telomeres, which are "the specific DNA-protein structures found at both ends of each chromosome," age quickly in these groups due to these stressors.[55] The result may be premature deaths and poorer health outcomes for groups that have been marginalized in our society owing to the rising prevalence of chronic diseases (obesity, cardiovascular disease, cancer, mental illness, diabetes), which are the responses to fatigued bodies from constant and aggressive stress experienced by racial and ethnic minorities and lower socioeconomic status individuals throughout history.

Recent research by the Federal Reserve Bank of Chicago examining the effects of the 1930s Home Owners' Loan Corporation policy by the Franklin D. Roosevelt administration, which led to redlining over two hundred cities across the United States, has also found significant impact from that 1930s' policy in communities today. Using a boundary design along with propensity score methods, researchers estimated the causal effects of the redlining maps on racial segregation, homeownership, house values, rents, and credit scores. They found that the policy had an "economically meaningful and lasting effect on the development of urban neighborhoods through reduced credit access and subsequent disinvestment."[56] It is not unreasonable to argue a strong connection between the stressors owing to current structural determinants, such as reduced credit access and subsequent community disinvestments among others, and past policies, such as the Home Owners' Loan Corporation Act that perpetuated the discriminatory and inequitable outcomes we see today. It is not an overstatement to conclude that the consequences of past policies continue to hurt disenfranchised groups of people, and legal and political remedies are necessary to correct the effects.

Second, the Supreme Court's statement on this issue, which is not supported by scientific evidence, has a rippling effect into other case law, thereby setting a precedent for other policies commissioned by other governmental bodies, which effectually enables averting responsibility and repairing the injustice. This recycling of poor arguments not only finds itself into other policies but also results in a similar attitude by other policy makers regarding whether and how to proceed with addressing inequities in our society. Ultimately, it equates to the policies that have been enacted and enforced versus those that have not been allowed to materialize and be fully implemented. This third point echoes the frustration of one of the most prominent health equity leaders in the United States, a former member of the US House of Representatives, Donna M. Christensen, MD, who stated: "One of the most disappointing revelations during my tenure in Congress has been the refusal by many lawmakers to follow or base our policies on what the science or research demonstrates. Instead they have based policies on politics, even though, ironically, the government is investing in research at the National Institutes of Health, Centers for Disease Control and Prevention, Agency for Healthcare Research and Quality, Substance Abuse and Mental Health Services Administration, and other agencies intended to strengthen the evidence-base for policy decisions."[57]

Third, the Supreme Court has been moving toward arbitrarily determining the point at which these vestiges of legally sanctioned discrimination cease to significantly impact certain communities, essentially arguing that after a certain time it does not matter anymore. If "reason" is the soul of all law, then it should be troubling that the court's unsubstantiated and fallacious arguments continue to stand despite evidence to the contrary. It is futile to make such arguments in the face of increasing research demonstrating the opposite conclusion and when considering the notion that we can draw a direct line from one law or policy after another to the impact they have today in terms of inequities.

Case after case and statute after statute through the centuries show justice's remarkable blindness, whether intentional or unintentional, to the structural racism and other forms of discrimination maintained and heightened in our society through law, "scientific" studies, and medicine. On March 6, 1857, the Supreme Court handed down its 7-2 decision in the Dred Scott case arguing that slaves were not citizens of the United States and therefore had no rights to sue in federal courts. Chief Justice Roger *current?*

Taney argued, "There are two clauses in the Constitution which point directly and specifically to the negro race as a separate class of persons, and show clearly that they were not regarded as a portion of the people or citizens of the Government then formed."

At the time, the majority of justices on the Supreme Court came from proslavery states or had connections to proslavery presidents. Eleven years later, in 1868, congressional members who were more enlightened and motivated to tackle the structural racism in some of our nation's major laws, passed the Fourteenth Amendment, which overturned the Dred Scott decision by granting citizenship to all those born in the United States, regardless of color. Unfortunately, this bold effort to stomp out racist laws and achieve equal protection for all groups was short-lived. It would be no match for opponents who were regrouping to employ various political determinants to maintain and worsen health inequities.

Despite slavery's existence in America for approximately 250 years before the Civil War ended, in 1883, less than two decades after slavery was abolished, the Supreme Court struck down the antidiscrimination provisions of the Civil Rights Act of 1875, arguing that eighteen years was enough time for African Americans to overcome the effects of slavery and get on their feet. The court reasoned, "When a man has emerged from slavery, there must be some stage in the progress of his elevation when he takes the rank of a mere citizen, and ceases to be the special favorite of the laws."[58] Notwithstanding the argument of which group of people were truly the "favorite of the laws," the court's arbitrary determination that eighteen years was sufficient to overcome the effects of slavery was not grounded in science or research. The court failed to understand slavery's biological and psychological implications on people for generations and the power of structural discrimination in our country. Immediately after the court struck down this antidiscrimination law, numerous laws were enacted around the country to further erode civil rights, voting rights, housing rights, and other critical protections for minority groups, which resulted in reducing the stage newly freed people had managed to reach during the eighteen years post–Civil War. Interestingly, these segregation-era laws bore a striking resemblance to laws that were first initiated in the thirteen original colonies, which further concretized the racial hierarchy that was first initiated in the 1600s.

More recently, in 2013, the Supreme Court once again used a similar argument to justify its decision to erode a federal law intended to protect

2013

minorities from discrimination. In *Shelby County v. Holder*, which was initiated during the wake of the most diverse Congress in US history, the Supreme Court overturned a key provision of the Voting Rights Act intended to protect against racial discrimination in voting. The court argued that current conditions at the time no longer warranted some aspects of the law[59] and further stated that "nearly 50 years later, things have changed dramatically. Largely because of the Voting Rights Act, '[v]oter turnout and registration rates' in covered jurisdictions 'now approach parity. Blatantly discriminatory evasions of federal decrees are rare. And minority candidates hold office at unprecedented levels.'" According to the Brennan Center for Justice, "Since the ruling, several states previously covered under preclearance moved to restrict voting rights. Since then, many states, including several previously covered by Section 5, ha[ve] moved to implement restrictive voting measures."

In other cases, including a case in 2016, the court has employed another argument to justify its reasoning that vestiges or past wrongs sanctioned by the state have no substantial impact today. This erroneous argument involves the notion that we are "rapidly becoming" an "integrated country" and that racial and ethnic prejudice is receding.[60] Clearly, the court has failed to appreciate the seriousness of these lingering and persistent vestiges of racism and other forms of discrimination and the detrimental impact they still have and will have in the future. Also clear is that the court has struggled to determine at what point the judicial branch should terminate interventions for certain groups, but it seems that as time passes it will become harder to convince this governmental body and others about the serious impact these vestiges of past wrongs still have on the health and well-being of certain groups. Instead, the court would rather view these inequities as products of "private choices" or products of social determinants so they do not have constitutional implications or legally enforceable remedies. Health equity advocates who continue to make the case that inequities are solely socially derived rather than politically derived will only bolster the Supreme Court's viewpoint, thus weakening legal protections to check these structural and institutional forms of discrimination as well as denying legal remedies to those impacted by inequities.

According to Professor Sidney Watson and Professor Ruqaiijah Yearby of Saint Louis University School of Law, structural discrimination advantages one group to the disadvantage of another, whereas institutional discrimination employs seemingly facially neutral policies that have a disparate impact on racial and ethnic groups, women, LGBTQ+ individuals, and people with disabilities, among others.[61] A modern example of structural discrimination involves the accessibility of health care, which is based on ability to pay. Under this system, more affluent individuals are structurally advantaged while lower socioeconomic status individuals are structurally disadvantaged because they are unable to pay for health services and may be diverted to health care providers based on their circumstances.

Juxtapose that to an example of institutional discrimination such as the Social Security Act's original exclusion of agricultural and domestic workers. These jobs were held largely by women and minorities, effectively leaving out almost half the working population. Or consider the three time periods in US history involving the opioid crisis and how criminal laws were developed depending on who was most impacted. When Chinese immigrants or African Americans were disproportionately impacted, the law was designed to punish, but when the crisis impacted whites, the laws were designed to be rehabilitative. These laws were institutionally discriminatory because they singled out opium (Chinese immigrants) versus heroin (whites) in the 1870s and crack (African Americans) versus cocaine (whites) in the 1970s and opioids (whites) in the 2000s.

Since housing is an essential determinant of health, a home buyer may experience additional structural barriers, making it difficult to access safe and affordable housing owing to past redlining practices by the government and commercial banks, which prohibited loans to certain communities and refused to insure loans for certain racial or immigrant groups, which led to racially segregated neighborhoods.[62] An example of institutional discrimination relative to housing occurs when zoning laws prevent the development of affordable housing units in certain neighborhoods to keep property values high and keep certain groups out. For such institutional discrimination, absent a legislative intent to discriminate against someone based on their race or national origin, the legal system refuses to apply its strictest scrutiny to such policies, unless there is a disparate impact. As a result, unless the government fails to provide a rational basis for enacting a policy, it is also challenging to overturn a facially neutral governmental decision or action.

Perhaps one of the earliest examples of structural discrimination involves the legal right to claim land ownership in the United States by European settlers who expelled Native Americans from their homes. Land ownership is one of the most important factors that impacts health status. James I, king of England, granted patent letters to English settlers arguing that Native Americans were "savages" and so through "conquest" European settlers were legally allowed to have titles for land transferred to them, an argument the US Supreme Court adopted in 1823 to deny Native Americans any claim to lands their forbears once held. This political action led to the westward expansion and settlement, "which history now reveals led to widespread dissemination of European-borne illnesses such as smallpox, measles, influenza, and other communicable diseases, also facilitated the decimation of millions of Native Americans who lacked immunological protection against foreign germs."[63]

Another example of structural discrimination includes the early colonial laws protecting slave owners' interests in slavery or legalizing slavery in the 1600s. New York became the first colony to establish a law forbidding its residents from harboring or feeding runaway slaves, followed by Massachusetts and Connecticut. Massachusetts became the first colony to legalize slavery in 1641, followed by Connecticut, Maryland, New York, New Jersey, the Carolinas, and Virginia. Throughout the 1600s and 1700s, the colonies passed other laws preventing enslaved individuals opportunities to overcome their state of affairs. Such laws included forbidding black people from bearing arms, congregating in large numbers, walking at night without passes or without lanterns, and keeping white servants (if the individuals were free blacks or Native Americans). Laws also acquitted slave masters of killing their slaves during punishment and mandated harsh punishment for slaves who assaulted Christians (whites) or attempted escape. Other laws during this time made it illegal for slaves to move abroad, raise food, earn money, and learn to read English, policies that forcefully reared their opportunistic heads repeatedly during the country's ensuing history. Consider, for example, constitutional negotiations that implicitly endorsed slavery with its Three-Fifths Compromise, Jim Crow laws during the post–Civil War segregation era, and other public policies intended to drive the status quo even into the present. The intentional concretization in laws and other policies of subjugating African slaves and Indians to unequal treatment has become so ingrained in our structures and institutions today that many people fail to see the cleverness of health equity opponents in systematically recycling many of these policy ideas and strategies over generations.

Why does this matter from a social determinants of health perspective? Because these policies still have far-reaching implications today. In 1963, Dr. Martin Luther King Jr. recognized

> there is a need to go for the *causal root*, to grapple with the problem at that point and to get rid of the notion once and for all that there are superior and inferior races. There are too many things alive in our nation and in our world to disprove this notion that has existed all too long. Then we're challenged after working in the realm of ideas, to move out into the arena of social action and to work passionately and unrelentingly to make racial justice a reality. In other words, there is great need to develop an action program in order to *remove all of the vestiges* of the old order.[64]

According to Richard Rothstein, author of *The Color of Law*, a seminal book on the US government's involvement in segregating America, "without our government's purposeful imposition of racial segregation, the other causes—private prejudice, white flight, real estate steering, bank redlining, income differences, and self-segregation—still would have existed but with far less opportunity for expression."[65] A similar argument could be made regarding the political determinants of health and other determinants of health, whereby inequities would still exist owing to social and other determinants of health, but the political determinants intensified their opportunity for expression. Once communities were starved of the resources they needed because of governmental policy, the commercial interests followed suit, wary of investing in those communities that the government had intentionally sidelined. Thus, the dearth of accessible quality health care providers, grocery stores, public transportation, educational facilities, and employment opportunities in many of these disparately treated communities, which, collectively, have prevented us from realizing health equity for all communities. Despite the US government's partial commitment to health equality over the past several decades with the advent of health laws such as the Hill-Burton Act, the Civil Rights Act of 1964, the Medicare and Medicaid law, the Children's Health Insurance Program, and the Affordable Care Act, unless we address the past policies that led to the inequities in our system and fully commit to comprehensively tackling inequities upstream in all areas from education to housing to transportation to employment among others that are structurally embedded in our society, and provide a legally enforceable mechanism to adjudicate such problems, we will make little progress in keeping the social determinants in check.

As we drill down to the interpersonal and intrapersonal levels, we see the force of law and public policies enabling both conscious and unconscious biases. Interpersonal discrimination is a more subtle form of prejudice that occurs at the individual level in social interactions, whereas intrapersonal discrimination involves implicit biases within an individual. A woman who has experienced a condescending clinician demonstrates the interplay between the social-ecological levels. The clinician's personal biases could represent interpersonal discrimination but is amplified to the structural level when you look at the power imbalances that give license to the clinician to behave with impunity. Research has shown clinicians have discriminated against certain groups of patients, including African Americans, Hispanics, and Native Americans, by not prescribing them needed medications for pain, amputating their extremities at higher rates for diabetes, and prejudging their ability to pay for care by not offering additional necessary health services. Other examples of interpersonal barriers that affect health outcomes and life expectancy include landlords refusing to rent to applicants with "ethnic"-sounding names, who are homosexual, or who have disabilities. According to Dr. Dayna Bowen Matthew, a leading scholar on bias at the University of Virginia, this form of discrimination, whether conscious or unconscious, has been enabled by the rule of law—a fact bolstered by the evidence presented earlier in this chapter.[66] In addition, intrapersonal barriers recognize that each individual is a product of his or her society and those who harbor unchecked prejudice will harm not only the victim but also the perpetrator. Sometimes advocates, individually, can be a barrier to advancing health equity.

Unless advocates and policy makers overcome these different levels of discrimination, they will be unable to advance their health equity agenda. Throughout America's history, these stubborn barriers have intentionally led to excluding certain groups from reaping the benefits of policies and programs or have disparately and negatively impacted a less powerful or privileged group. Because of these barriers, the United States has only instituted a few public policies or initiatives focused on bolstering health equity for all groups, which has resulted in many groups being unable to fully contribute to the enhancement of our society.

The third major political determinant of health—policy—provides a number of tools that have been used to overcome past barriers and may be helpful in the future with expected demographic changes sure to exacerbate inequities if left unchecked. If the political determinants of health continue to exclude certain groups from fully participating and benefiting from the country's resources, which are critical to attaining optimal health, the result will be a tremendous economic burden and a weakening of the country's national security. Fewer healthy people means fewer people gaining the skills and education to work or serve in the military, which means fewer people contributing to the tax base and helping to improve and expand our infrastructure or defend the nation from threats. Advocates should note, however, that expected demographic changes may undo many of the gains achieved through leveraging the political determinants of health throughout the decades. The unraveling of gains is based on arguments raised by Supreme Court justices who have been wary of policies and programs intended to help one historically marginalized group catch up educationally and otherwise as well as the court's consistent efforts to systematically and surgically weaken existing laws that affect the rules of politics.

The Third Political Determinant of Health: Policy

Policy, the third political determinant of health, cements government decisions and is defined as a law, a regulation, a procedure, an administrative action, a plan, an incentive, or a voluntary practice of government undertaken to achieve specific health goals within a society. According the World Health Organization, "an explicit health policy can achieve several things: it defines a vision for the future which in turn helps to establish targets and points of reference for the short and medium term. It outlines priorities and the expected roles of different groups; and it builds consensus and informs people."[67] In addition, it provides a mechanism to enforce rights that have been gained or challenge those that deny rights. Of course, this political determinant of health is not a be-all-end-all; it is another mechanism that can help advocates achieve greater traction in their efforts to advance health equity. Advocates should keep in mind that, while they may have realized success on this front, there are usually efforts under way to leverage the first two political determinants of health—voting and government—to void the results achieved in the third political determinant of health, policy.

To realize any significant headway with political determinants of health, the stars have to align perfectly. As we will later see, elections

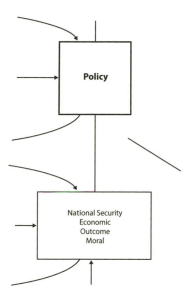

Policy as a political determinant of health.

may produce a majority of decision makers sensitive to a particular issue, but without advocates' continued, determined efforts on the outside once the government convenes, the particular issue will likely never be addressed. Sometimes a bill can get through a legislature and be vetoed by the president or governor, or a bill can even be enacted and then fail to be implemented or enforced by successive administrations. Sometimes a bill can be signed into law by a president or a governor and upheld by successive administrations, but then a court overturns the law. Or a state government may decide not to adopt, participate in, or implement a federal policy, as when Congress passed the Excellence in Mental Health Act[68] after advocates expended considerable time, energy, and resources to secure its passage. The policy's purpose was to increase access to community-based behavioral health services for mental health and substance use treatments and to improve Medicaid reimbursement for those services, but some states refused to participate.

Same Framework → Different Strategy → Similar Goal (End)

As health equity advocates move forward with their agenda to develop and implement policy, they should keep in mind that both

Republicans and Democrats are driven by a need to make change to safe-guard the present and future of the country. Often policy makers from both sides of the aisle have referenced the same framework as the foundations for their policy making, such as Maslow's hierarchy of needs, McKinlay's population health model, McLeroy's social ecological model, or the Institute for Healthcare Improvement's Triple Aim. However, there is a fundamental difference in strategy and approach. With this in mind, there are four arguments that have been tried and proved effective across the political spectrum to elevate or to undermine efforts to overcome the structural, institutional, interpersonal, and intrapersonal barriers that prevent us from prioritizing health equity in policy: moral, performance, economic, and national security arguments.

In the United States, a progression of categorical arguments to elevate health equity for vulnerable groups have resonated with Democrats, Republicans, and Independents. First is the moral argument, which is steeped in Judeo-Christian principles and was used to argue for abolishing slavery and to afford enslaved individuals and other marginalized groups quality health services and supports. Second is the performance, or outcomes, argument, which was used to pass educational reforms such as No Child Left Behind. Third is the economic argument, which was used in support of providing health care access to sailors who were deemed vital to trade. Fourth is the national security argument, which was used to convince federal policy makers to establish a national institute to research mental illness because too many young adults were deemed unfit for military service. (To more fully understand how these arguments have effectively or ineffectively been used in the United States, see chapter 2.)

Despite some efforts to advance health equity in America via policy, usually health equity proponents have found themselves working to overcome policy interventions aimed at making it more difficult for groups without power and privilege to engage in the process. For health equity proponents, policy interventions usually present more challenges, but for health equity opponents, these interventions provide opportunities to maintain the status quo and thwart efforts to advance a health equity agenda. That is why understanding how proponents and opponents have leveraged policy interventions for their agendas warrants a closer look.

The Grassroots: Advocacy

At the heart of the health equity movement are health equity proponents who must directly act to address the ramifications of the po-

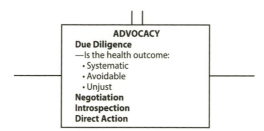

Key advocacy elements for addressing the political determinants of health.

litical determinants of health. They must connect the dots for stakeholders that show how voting, government, and policy impact our ability to lead healthy and quality lives and how these political determinants of health interventions have prevented us from achieving health equity for individuals living in the United States. It is, therefore, crucial not to leave it up to trust because government is a human institution where individuals are making the decisions and are responsible for its evolution. Those closest to the policy move the infrastructure forward, which is why people matter.

Successful advocacy entails completing several phases. As Martin Luther King Jr. recognized during the civil rights movement, there are four phases to advocacy that apply even today to support efforts to bolster health equity at the grassroots level. These include (1) conducting due diligence to systematically ascertain whether inequities exist; (2) researching, exploring, and negotiating possible solutions; (3) engaging in the inventory process of introspection to determine personal and organizational strengths and weaknesses; and (4) acting to enable, to prioritize, and to enforce opportunities to create and advance health equity in communities.[69]

During the due diligence phase, three factors determine whether an inequity exists as noted by Dr. Paula Braveman at the University of California, San Francisco, and other notable experts at the World Health Organization.[70] First, is the difference in health outcomes systematic, systemic, or both? Second, is the difference in health outcomes avoidable? Third, is the difference in health outcomes unjust? After determining whether an inequity exists and to what extent, one should then conduct the necessary research to understand its origins, including its historical and political roots, and employ an ecological approach to address the problem to better inform the advocacy strategy. At the same time, it is important to engage in the collaborative and community-led process of exploring and negotiating the best solutions at various levels for the affected community, remembering to consider the commercial interests and the government investment value that may be impacted as well as how they may be leveraged. And equally important, strategically think about both the governmental and the nongovernmental partners who should be engaged in your effort.

Once the due diligence and negotiation phases have been completed, then the next phase involves introspection to prepare the individual, community, organization, or coalition for direct action in the political process. Complete an action plan during this phase with input from all interested stakeholders. Also during this phase, commitments from potential strategic partners must be secured and responsibilities finalized before directly engaging in the advocacy process.

After the three initial advocacy phases have occurred, a fourth phase involves direct action to address the ramifications of the political determinants of health: voting, government, and policy. This phase involves targeting interventions and resources to address the needs of populations who find themselves in detrimental life situations, thereby enabling opportunities to advance health equity. Each political determinant of health provides opportunities for advocates to initiate legally enforceable changes and allocate resources that improve the conditions of daily living.

One could leverage elections (voting) to introduce and pass citizen-initiated ballot measures or legislatively referred ballot measures, such as expanding Medicaid, expanding mental health services, requiring dialysis centers to refund money to insurers or patients, enforcing a new ratio of nurses to patients in some hospital facilities, or banning local governments from enacting soda taxes. All of these measures have been attempted. In addition to recruiting and electing the power brokers who fill roles in government crucial to advancing health equity initiatives, one could also use this opportunity to highlight health inequities plaguing a community and generate ideas that the government should be interested in addressing once it is formally organized and authorized to do so.

One could leverage government, which determines whether and to what extent it will allow policies to advance or be enforced, which has serious implications for health equity. On one extreme end of the spectrum, health equity might not only be stalled but also pushed back to the point where it would take thousands of years to realize when governments fail to advance or enforce policies. Such is the case in California concerning affordable housing with a fifty-year-old state housing law intended to bolster affordable housing development.[71] The law requires local governments to examine the number of permits they issue for building housing at various income levels and produce reports on their progress. However, the state government did not hold these local governments accountable for not producing these reports, much less meet their housing goals.[72] In 2017, state government officials were not sure whether cities and counties had met their housing goals nor was there any "reliable measure of how many houses are being built in California for low-, middle- and upper-income residents," according to the *Los Angeles Times*.[73] Without continued and effective advocacy to monitor progress, to remind government officials of the government's investment value in enforcing this law, and to be accountable on the policy, it has set back the attainment of health equity relative to housing affordability for generations to come.

Juxtapose that result with a more recent issue involving the federal health reform law, the Affordable Care Act, where there was continued strong and effective advocacy to prevent the invalidation of the law and thus preserve opportunities to advance and realize health equity much sooner. Almost ten years after the law was enacted, evidence showed that, with just Medicaid expansion alone, there had been a significant increase in access to substance use treatment,[74] improvement in colon cancer survival,[75] and better cardiac mortality.[76] Notwithstanding these positive outcomes, in December 2018, a federal district court judge in Texas issued a sweeping decision that a key provision of the Affordable Care Act—the individual mandate requiring most people to have health insurance—is unconstitutional since Congress zeroed out the penalty. He ruled that the entire health law should be invalidated as a result, including the health equity-focused provisions of the law. Immediately after this ruling was published, the US Department of Health and Human Services issued a statement to underscore that it would "continue administering and enforcing all aspects of the ACA as it had before the court issued its decision. This decision does not require that Health and Human Services make any changes to ACA programs it administers or its enforcement of any portion of the ACA at this time."[77] Interestingly, after coming out of an election season in which health care was, for the first time in US history, the number one concern for voters, the Department of Health and

Human Services recognized the political disaster the judge's ruling would create and tried to get ahead of it. In this example, advocates leveraged the 2018 midterm elections to raise health care issues as their biggest priority, and although their efforts helped to pass state health care-related ballot initiatives across the country, their efforts also helped to ensure that the federal government did not completely undermine gains made in advancing health equity under the health reform law.

In addition to leveraging the elections and government to advance health equity agendas, one could also leverage policy to fund research or programs that directly address health inequities, such as the Centers for Disease Control and Prevention's Racial and Ethnic Approaches to Community Health (REACH) program, or prohibit the funding of research or programs that consequentially create or exacerbate inequities. More often, health equity proponents may find themselves being less proactive and more reactive. In the past, these advocates unsuccessfully tried many times to move a policy idea over the finish line, but they had to refocus their attention when opponents tried to undermine existing policies, for example, when opponents successfully pushed for a policy rider or amendment prohibiting federal funding from being used to sponsor gun-violence research in 1996. More disappointing is the fact that once a health equity-focused policy has been repealed, it has usually taken generations to resurrect that policy.

At each recurrent and critical stage of the political process, health equity advocates are faced with opportunities to move the agenda forward or protect it from being undermined. Having enough or the right policies is never sufficient. Advocacy is a multifaceted and continual process at every level of the political spectrum. It does not end once a policy is achieved in any given branch of government or even among all branches of government, because the political pendulum always swings back and forth as Dr. Alpha Bryan, the executive director of the Clayton County Board of Health in Georgia, has recognized working in a government health agency.[78]

Advocacy is a complex and time-consuming process that can take countless hours, days, weeks, and even years of sacrifice and hard work, which is why President Bill Clinton once acknowledged in a speech to college students, "I think that it's very important to understand we live in a time when, for a whole variety of reasons, policy making tends to be dimly understood, often distrusted and disconnected from the consequences of the policies being implemented."[79] Advocates must understand the role the political determinants of health play to leverage them to tackle health inequities. Chapter 4 provides a deeper dive into advocacy surrounding the Obama administration's health reform efforts, which incorporated the most robust health equity agenda in public policy and law. It is intended to show how this model could be used by health equity advocates in the future.

4

How the Game Is Played
Successful Employment of the Political Determinants of Health

No one really knows how the game is played
The art of the trade
How the sausage gets made. . . .
No one really knows how the
Parties get to yes
The pieces that are sacrificed in
Ev'ry game of chess
—Lin-Manuel Miranda, "The Room Where It Happens"

The political determinants of health have long been used to prevent the prioritization of health equity in America, but very few people understand how the political game is played and how the "sausage" or policy gets made. US Supreme Court Justice Sandra Day O'Connor acknowledged this point: "We have a complex system of government. You have to teach it to every generation."[1] Even with the few instances when proponents of health equity successfully leveraged the political determinants of health to increase opportunities to advance health equity, not many people are familiar with how those results were accomplished. Chapters 4 and 5 highlight one of those few times that advocates succeeded in prioritizing and passing a major policy focused on bolstering health equity, namely, the Affordable Care Act. These chapters will focus on the strategies and tactics employed to ultimately produce and pass the most robust and inclusive federal health policy to advance health equity in the United States.

Senator Paul Wellstone once declared, "There are three critical ingredients to democratic renewal and progressive change in America: good public policy, grassroots organizing and electoral politics."[2] Chapters 4 and 5 will underscore not only how voting, government, and policy changes affected the creation and evolution of the Affordable Care Act and other health policies but also how grassroots organizing was strategically employed to advance public initiatives that prioritized health equity for all population groups in the United States.

The Beginning of Change: Voting

The year 2008 was an exhilarating time to be involved in health equity advocacy. Presidential elections were taking place in November, and health reform was proving to be a major campaign issue for both Democrats and Republicans. Republican presidential candidate John McCain proposed improving the quality of health insurance through competition. McCain's plan would provide individuals with tax credits to purchase insurance and loosen state rules governing the sale of insurance by allowing people to buy policies across state lines. Though he opposed federally mandated universal coverage, McCain was the first candidate to endorse the use of universal tax credits to provide access to private health insurance.[3] Republican candidate Mitt Romney also endorsed a system of tax deductions to help individuals buy insurance. Romney, despite having enacted universal coverage in Massachusetts when he was governor, disavowed national mandated coverage. He proposed allowing states to devise their own insurance plans and providing states with financial incentives to deregulate their health insurance markets.

The Republican primaries were short-lived, with John McCain securing the nomination by March 2008. By contrast, the Democratic primary contest ran well into the summer. The final two candidates, Barack Obama and Hillary Clinton, both listed health reform as a major priority and endorsed proposals seeking to make health insurance affordable for all Americans. Unlike the Republican proposals, which emphasized using market competition to control health care costs, the Democratic candidates sought to increase the government's involvement in the health care system. Both candidates' proposals provided for government-offered insurance plans; however, while Clinton's plan would require that everyone have insurance, Obama's plan did not.

Both candidates also would prevent private insurers from denying health insurance on the basis of preexisting conditions—an issue that resonated with millions of Americans. Preexisting conditions hit close to home for many families who struggled to get affordable health coverage. Whether McCain or one of the two remaining Democratic candidates won the election, it was clear that some kind of health reform package was possible with the next administration. Health equity proponents sprang into action to meet with officials from both Democratic and Republican campaigns to educate them about health inequities and to urge them to prioritize health equity in their health reform proposals. Past failures at passing health reform did not mean it was impossible to achieve this feat, and health equity proponents were convinced that with demographic shifts, increasing health care costs, and out-of-reach and out-of-sight health care access, it was an opportune time to push the agenda forward. This was the atmosphere at the time, the potential for sweeping reform, and health equity advocates knew major changes were ahead.

Perhaps even more exciting for health equity advocates was the recognition that this was a rare opportunity. They leveraged the moment to push their agenda, scoring an important win. For the first time in American history, they had convinced a presidential candidate, Obama, to explicitly include the elimination of racial and ethnic health disparities as a key health policy priority for his health reform agenda during the campaign and helped to garner the support he needed to win the election. After the election, this commitment to health equity and eliminating health disparities was broadened to include other forms of disparities among people with disabilities, LGBTQ+ individuals, veterans, women, and older adults.

The possibility of comprehensive health reform and health equity-focused policies became evident when the Senate Finance Committee on May 6, 2008, under the leadership of Max Baucus (D-MT), held the first in a series of hearings on health reform during the second session of the 110th Congress. The hearing titled *Seizing the New Opportunity for Health Reform* coincided with the 2008 presidential campaigns and would take place into the next year, when the 111th Congress would more than likely be tackling these issues. The hearings would lay the foundation for developing policy and building consensus "on how to provide access to affordable high-quality health care for all Americans." Unlike in 1993, when Senate Finance Committee chair Daniel Patrick Moynihan (D-NY) was not particularly enthusiastic about health reform, Baucus expressed confidence that, this time around, he and his colleagues would succeed in passing a health reform bill.

During the hearings, Baucus underscored that the issues impacting the health care system had become unmanageable, the incremental or piecemeal solutions Congress had employed to date were simply inadequate, and the problems would only get worse before they got better unless Congress meaningfully addressed them. From his standpoint, the moral and economic argument for health reform had never been stronger, and the health reform proposals that had been developed by both Democrats and Republicans over the decades showed striking similarities and shared principles. These similarities included universal health coverage, greater protections for consumers and providers, value-based purchasing, comparative effectiveness research, and greater use of health information technology and electronic health records.

Baucus believed that the opportunity was ripe, since it was increasingly evident there was unprecedented eagerness to work together to fix these problems in their health care and public health systems among major health care stakeholders, interest groups, coalitions, and even presidential candidates. He did, however, recognize the challenges that were ahead despite these significant gains in consensus. The committee would have to resolve key issues, such as whether to mandate health insurance coverage, how to finance universal health insurance coverage, and what roles the federal government, state governments, employers, and families should play.

Senator Chuck Grassley (R-IA), the ranking member of the committee, also acknowledged the growing and costly problem of uninsurance in the United States—how difficult it was for many Americans to access affordable coverage. Just like Baucus, Grassley recognized that the incremental solutions Congress had initiated to date were not effective in curbing health care costs. He believed that private market solutions were the best route and issued a warning to the committee about not repeating past mistakes or disrupting the system too much:

> It makes the most sense to build on the private health insurance system. As you all know, people are used to their employer providing health benefits. They like their employers' work and they do not want us to disturb that. They like that their employers take care of their billing, and by and large they are satisfied. They learned 14 years ago during the Clinton health plan debate that, even in the midst of call for change, many people like what they have. So health reform should not up-end the system and do harm while trying to help folks without insurance. I also think they need to be prudent in taking on new obligations through government.[4]

Grassley warned that any health reform package must be bipartisan and should have broad support among the American people. He stated that, although these were "tough policy problems," he was "encouraged that the issue is back on the table."[5]

At the hearing, ideas were solicited from two former secretaries of the Department of Health and Human Services, Donna Shalala from the Clinton administration and Tommy Thompson from the Bush administration. Shalala emphasized the areas of consensus between both sides that Baucus had outlined earlier, which included addressing the health workforce issue. She echoed Grassley's warning about exercising care when developing a bill that would impact virtually everyone—a lesson she had learned in 1993. Shalala also urged the committee to reach consensus on not only the problem but also the solutions.

Thompson also used his time to emphasize the need for health reform to reduce costs and to accomplish this in a bipartisan manner. Like Baucus, he recognized that all three presidential candidates had elevated health reform in their campaigns and urged the next president of the United States to convene a commission with an equal number of Republicans and Democrats to offer recommendations for health reform. Interestingly, Thompson was the first in the hearing to emphasize the need to address wellness and prevention of chronic disease in a health reform bill—moving from a disease system to a wellness system. He was also the first person to mention the urgent need to address racial and ethnic health disparities. "But there are ways in which they can get information out on nutrition, which they really have to do, especially with minorities," he said. "Being overweight leads into diabetes, which is an epidemic in Native Americans, Latinos, and African Americans. *They have to do something about it.*"[6]

After this hearing, House and Senate committee chairs and their staff who had jurisdiction over health care issues convened informal discussions and strategic planning around health reform. When it became apparent that these discussions were taking place, health equity advocates knew this was an opportunity they had to seize immediately. Taking Thompson's words to heart, they were convinced it was time to take action to inform lawmakers about the health policy issues impacting vulnerable and underserved communities in the United States.

Senator Edward M. Kennedy, who chaired the Senate Health, Education, Labor and Pensions Committee, had been recently diagnosed with a malignant brain tumor and required aggressive treatments. Kennedy had dedicated much of his career to ensuring that all Americans had access to high-quality, affordable health care, and in speaking of health reform in *Newsweek*, he said, "This is the cause of my life." In 1971, Kennedy became the chair of the Senate Health Subcommittee and began his campaign for national health insurance. Among the many landmark laws enacted under his leadership and sponsorship over the years were the Protection and Advocacy for Mentally Ill Individuals Act of 1986, the Americans with Disabilities Act of 1990, the Ryan White Comprehensive AIDS Resources Emergency Act of 1990, the National Institutes of Health Revitalization Act of 1993, the Health Insurance Portability and Accountability Act of 1996, the Mental Health Parity Act of 1996, and the creation of the State Children's Health Insurance Program in 1997. Despite his illness, Kennedy declared his commitment to realizing health reform once and for all: "I am resolved to see to it this year that they create a system to ensure that someday, when there is a cure for the disease I now have, no American who needs it will be denied it."[7]

Amid this upheaval in the health policy arena, a major news story broke that brought the issue of health disparities to light in a tragic way. Esmin Green, a forty-nine-year-old African American woman, had been brought to the emergency room of a local hospital on the morning of June 18, 2008. Hospital records stated that she was exhibiting agitation and psychosis and was involuntarily admitted after refusing treatment. During the first week of July, major news media outlets aired a video showing Green sitting in a waiting room at a hospital in New York for nearly twenty-four hours and then collapsing from her chair. Once she collapsed, neither fellow patients nor the hospital's staff moved to help her, even as she writhed on the floor trying to get up. Two security guards and a member of the hospital's medical staff could be seen on the video, briefly stopping to look at Green before walking away. She stopped moving roughly thirty minutes after falling and was dead when a nurse finally examined her another thirty minutes after that. According to the medical examiner, she had died after developing blood clots in her legs from the long period of physical inactivity.[8] The widespread outcry from the public spurred health equity advocates into action and provided a vivid and tragic example of the results of health disparities.

Despite the major media attention around disparate treatment at the time and the broad health reform principles that both the Democratic and Republican candidates had promulgated, addressing health disparities did not seem to be "a priority issue in the 2008 election."[9] However, unlike McCain's proposal, which included provisions that would implicitly address health disparities, Obama's proposal explicitly aimed to address their root causes. Obama's proposal included language that would prioritize data collection on disparate populations' access to quality care, increasing the diversity of the health workforce, ensuring cultural competence, and improving the capacity of safety-net institutions.[10] Whichever candidate won the presidential election, health equity proponents knew Thompson was right—they had to do something to address health disparities and prioritize health equity before health reform negotiations picked up full speed in the new year.

The Turning Point: Leveraging Government to Create a More Inclusive and Equitable Health Law

In November 2008, Obama was elected the forty-fourth president of the United States. Health reform had been a major part of his campaign platform, and he proposed a significant overhaul of the health care system. Among many other changes, his Plan for a Healthy America would create a new federal health plan, or public option, for the uninsured, providing benefits comparable to those offered to federal employees, and establish a national health insurance exchange where individuals would be able to select the public plan or an approved private plan.[11] Premiums would be subsidized for low-income and middle-class individuals and families. Insurance companies would be prohibited from denying coverage on the basis of illness or preexisting conditions, and insurance coverage would be mandated for children. Prevention and public health as well as the adoption and use of health information technology were also a cornerstone of his health reform proposal. After the elections, it was interesting to watch the convergence of all three major presidential candidates' health reform ideas morphing into what would later become the Affordable Care Act, or ObamaCare.

Although President Obama produced and promulgated an outline of his health reform priorities, Congress was charged with building on those priorities and determining the scope of the health reform package. The Senate Finance Committee operated with lightning speed and only eight days after the presidential election, on November 12, 2008, produced a white paper—*Call to Action: Health Reform 2009*—which served as a blueprint for comprehensive health reform. In the paper, Baucus, the chair of the Senate Finance Committee, stated, "It is the duty of the next Congress to reform America's health care system."[12] This helped to lay the foundation for major changes to the health care system under the Obama administration.

Once the Obama-Biden transition team was in place, numerous organizations and health care stakeholders began to share their ideas for health reform, which helped White House officials get a better sense of what external advocacy groups wanted to see in a health reform bill. Health equity proponents from various organizations also voiced their concerns and shared their policy recommendations during the transition period. Some even shared their hopes and concerns for health reform publicly, including Congresswoman Hilda Solis (D-CA) and Dr. Brian Smedley, who participated in a Kaiser Family Foundation webcast in December 2008.[13] They voiced their hope that health reform would prioritize health equity, as Obama had promised when he was campaigning.

After the presidential election in 2008 and after the transition of administrations, Vice President Joe Biden suggested that the president should reconsider tackling health reform so early on in his administration. He was afraid that attempting to enact sweeping health reform might jeopardize the president's reelection. The nation was then in the midst of a major recession and crippling job losses, and Biden thought that the Obama administration should focus on creating jobs instead. He suggested this approach even though congressional leaders had already been holding meetings and hearings exploring this issue. Obama disagreed with the vice president, however, and decided to move forward. He believed that comprehensive health reform would help to create new jobs and stimulate the economy. Later on, at the American Medical Association's annual conference on June 15, 2009, the president made an economic and national security argument for health reform: "Make no mistake: The cost of our health care is a threat to our economy. It's an escalating burden on our families and businesses. It's a ticking time bomb for the federal budget. And it is unsustainable for the United States of America."[14] The president decided to risk losing his own reelection and the Democratic majorities in both chambers of Congress.

In addition to the historic election of the nation's first African American president, the House of Representatives had selected its first female Speaker of the House, Nancy Pelosi (D-CA), during the previous Congress. Pelosi had long championed efforts to increase access to health care and worked closely with Senator Harry Reid (D-NV) and the congressional Tri-Caucus to address health disparities. She once revealed that health reform was one of the pillars of who she was and later admitted, "I knew I came [to Congress] to vote for health care for all Americans."[15] She wasted no time naming the new chairs for the various committees in the House. Once those names were revealed, health reform advocates were hopeful that a comprehensive health reform bill was possible, one that would be broad and inclusive of a health equity agenda.

In a speech to a joint session of Congress on February 24, 2009, Obama urged lawmakers to move forward with health reform: "The cost of health care has weighed down their economy and their conscience long enough. So let there be no doubt, health care reform cannot wait, it must not wait and it will not wait another year."[16] As he did during his election campaign, the president underscored the increasing number of uninsured Americans and rapidly rising premiums, pledging to make changes that would both bring down costs and save lives. That month, serious negotiations over several health reform proposals were taking place in key committees of the House and Senate, namely, the Senate Health, Education, Labor and Pensions Committee led by Kennedy; the Senate Finance Committee led by Baucus; the House Energy and Commerce Committee led by Henry Waxman (D-CA); the House Ways and Means Committee led by Charles Rangel (D-NY); and the House Education and Labor Committee led by George Miller (D-CA). Clearly, health reform was going to take place, and soon. The leaders were showing unprecedented unity and an eagerness to cooperate to realize the ultimate goal that had escaped Congress and White House administrations through the decades.

Health equity advocates realized that this was another rare opportunity to advance a health equity agenda and address health disparities once and for all in a more comprehensive manner. However, health equity advocacy coalitions and organizations were not well coordinated, collaborative, or consistent in their legislative requests. Some advocates were focused only on health care quality improvement, some were focused primarily on data collection and reporting, and others were focused primarily on health workforce development, prevention and wellness, or language access. The disorganization among health equity advocates weakened the argument for including robust health equity provisions in the legislation.

Drafters of the health reform legislative proposals were uncertain where to seek counsel and whose priorities to include. They wanted assurance that any language submitted by advocates had been properly vetted and agreed on by the majority of stakeholders. And with the community disorganized and focused on competing goals, drafters were hesitant to help advocates. Consequently, the need to unite and mobilize, to streamline efforts, and to create a one-stop shop for information sharing and collaboration became increasingly important if health equity advocates wanted to be effective in realizing their goals.

The likelihood of health reform became even clearer to advocates during the first week of March when Obama announced the appointment of Kathleen Sebelius as secretary of the Department of Health and Human Services and Nancy-Ann DeParle as director of the White House Office of Health Reform. In remarks given on March 2, 2009, the president publicly recognized the success his administration had already achieved by advancing health reform through the American Recovery and Reinvestment Act. "They have done more to advance the cause of Health Care Reform in the last month than they have in the last decade."[17]

The stimulus law, which the act is often called, did, in fact, include provisions that laid the foundation for comprehensive health reform. It included investments in comparative effectiveness research, health workforce development, public health, and incentivizing providers to adopt and meaningfully use health information technology, most of which Obama had championed during his campaign. The president could have stopped there and argued that he did, in fact, fulfill his campaign promise, but he did not. He went on to urge the passage of a comprehensive bill that included critical health insurance reforms, delivery system reforms, and payment system reforms.

Three days after this announcement, on March 5, 2009, the White House convened a special four-hour summit on health care reform, inviting approximately 150 congressional and executive branch officials and other health policy experts to start serious deliberations on the issue. More than fifty members of Congress attended the event, including Speaker Nancy Pelosi, Congresswoman Donna Christensen, Congresswoman Jan Schakowsky, Congresswoman Allyson Schwartz, Senator Max Baucus, Senator Ted Kennedy, Senator Tom Harkin, Senator Sheldon Whitehouse, Senator Orrin Hatch, Senator Mike Enzi, Congressman Eric Cantor, and Senator Mitch McConnell.

A wide range of stakeholders and community leaders also attended, including representatives from AARP, the American Medical Association, the American Heart Association, the American Hospital Association, Planned Parenthood, the National Medical Association, the American Cancer Society, the National Minority AIDS Council, the Service Employees International Union, and the US Chamber of Commerce. Interestingly, many of the same people and organizations that had waged an aggressive campaign against health reform attempts under the Clinton administration now professed their interest in achieving health reform this time around. Physicians groups, nurses groups, hospital groups, labor unions, small and big businesses, and health insurance groups all echoed their readiness to be active and constructive participants in the process.

Opening the summit in the East Room, Melody Barnes, the White House's director of the Domestic Policy Council, introduced a firefighter who had heeded the president's call to organize a community discussion about health care back in December 2008. He presented a compilation of information, suggestions, and feedback from this effort. During the program, the president also gave remarks: "Their goal will be to enact comprehensive health reform by the end of this year."[18] In breakout sessions afterward, both Republican and Democratic lawmakers repeatedly stated that Congress needed to put politics aside and get health reform done as well as expressed their optimism that this Congress could succeed.

While attending the special forum, Christensen and another nongovernmental health equity advocate urged the president to ensure that the elimination of racial and ethnic health disparities was prioritized in health reform. Obama agreed that this was a serious issue that should be addressed in health reform, and, for the first time since becoming president, Obama publicly acknowledged support for including a health equity agenda in the law. At the same time, the White House was doing its part to advance ideas around health reform; negotiations were getting more serious in the Senate. Following the lead of the White House, the Senate Health, Education, Labor and Pensions (HELP) Committee held a stakeholders meeting on March 12, 2009, to provide updates on health reform efforts and continue the momentum initiated by the administration.

Seizing the Opportunity: Creating a Drumbeat across America

Without that outside drumbeat and outside mobilization, it is impossible for us to do the inside maneuvering to get the votes out to pass a bill.—*House Speaker Nancy Pelosi to advocates for health reform*

While these activities were ramping up in the White House and in the Senate, health reform advocates were proceeding with their advocacy efforts. After former First Lady Rosalynn Carter's annual mental health symposium in Atlanta, Georgia, on November 20, 2008, that year titled "Unclaimed Children Revisited: Fostering a Climate to Improve Children's Mental Health," a nongovernmental landmark report was released concerning the children's mental health system. The report showed that the needs of children and youth with mental health conditions were not being adequately addressed. The report provided guidance and impetus for improving mental health policies on a national level.[19]

Carter, along with other mental health champions, believed that this was a great opportunity to push forward mental health priorities for children, and so they convened an ad hoc group to discuss the issue and strategize about how best to proceed. Their group thought an appropriate strategy should include outreach to the Congressional Children's Caucus. So, they drafted and sent a letter to Congresswoman Sheila Jackson Lee, who was chairing the caucus at the time, urging her support for improving the children's mental health system and providing specific policy recommendations for developing a comprehensive public health framework for children and adolescent mental health.

They had started their advocacy in isolation, focusing primarily on children's mental and behavioral health issues, but health equity proponents soon realized that they could be more effective if they joined with other groups that shared their larger goal of advancing a health equity agenda. While health equity proponents were strategizing, the Los Angeles-based National Health Equity Coalition was in preliminary discussions with almost fifty organizations about creating a national campaign to interject the elimination of health disparities into national policy. Some individuals, however, were concerned about the use of the term *campaign*, arguing that it sounded more short term or narrowly focused or implied that the goals of their effort had already been established. They were concerned that other organizations interested in joining them would perceive that they would not have a say over shaping the activities of the group. Others argued for establishing a coalition to bring organizations together and create unity around a common cause.

While the National Health Equity Coalition was strategizing, one major health reform advocacy group, Health Care for America Now, was also forming a health disparities working group. Community Catalyst was interested in forming a similar group as well. Other groups representing disability advocates, LGBTQ+ advocates, women's advocates, rural advocates, and advocates of older adults were also forming their own coalitions to address disparities in health status among their respective populations. Various advocates among them started worrying that these efforts would actually undermine the overall goal of igniting a push for health equity in health reform negotiations. They were concerned about being overwhelmed with meetings and argued for better coordination of these groups since their agendas, missions, and goals seemed remarkably similar. Congressional staff, once again, worried about the impact these independent, competing campaigns would have or how effective they would be.

A single umbrella group was needed to serve as a point of contact to health reformers in Congress and the White House on health equity priorities. This was necessary to resolve conflicts, steer the strategy, initiate actions, build consensus, and develop vetted legislative language for inclusion in health reform bills. While all of these groups were creating coalitions or discussing how best to proceed, one thing was for sure: advocates recognized that health equity and the elimination of health disparities were not being addressed at all during health reform negotiations. A few weeks later, the children's mental health ad hoc group decided to broaden the scope of its advocacy to focus more broadly on health equity among all vulnerable populations and agreed to form a working group whose primary purpose would be to spearhead and coordinate advocacy to include robust health equity provisions in health reform proposals. That way they would not disrupt newly formed coalitions but, instead, serve as a convener or collaborative for all of these organizations.

This idea came out of prior lessons learned while working on the Mental Health Parity Act and the Americans with Disabilities Act Amendments Act on the Senate HELP Committee in 2007. Together with advocates who helped to spearhead those efforts, health equity proponents invited any coalitions or interested stakeholders to a meeting hosted by the American Psychological Association, which generously allowed this new group to leverage the organization's resources for this initiative. On April 1, 2009, health equity advocates invited people representing various health care stakeholders from mental and behavioral health, civil rights, women's rights, faith-based, disability, rural, providers, consumers, and LGBTQ+ organizations to join them in a serious dialogue on ensuring the prioritization of health equity in reform legislation.

The turnout on the day of the meeting was bigger than they expected and far more diverse. Instead of mainly groups or individuals focused on racial and ethnic issues, there were attendees from prominent groups with a broader health focus, such as the American Academy of Pediatrics, American Hospital Association, National Association of Public Hospitals and Health Systems (now known as America's Essential Hospitals), American Association of Marriage and Family Therapists, American Cancer Society Cancer Action Network, Families USA, America's Health Insurance Plans, American Public Health Association, Asian & Pacific Islander American Health Forum, National Association of Social Workers, the American Dental Association, the National Black Nurses Association, National Dental Association, the National Medical Association, National Hispanic Medical Association, National Immigration Law Center, AIDS Action, Child Welfare League of America, First Focus, National Association of Community Health Centers, National Urban League, NAACP, National Health Law Program, National Partnership for Women and Families, Japanese American Citizens League, National Alliance for Hispanic Health, National Coalition for LGBT Health, Hispanic Federation, and Society for Public Health Education. They were excited to see organizations as well as coalitions coming together to share information and strategies to advance the discussion.

During the meeting, advocates explained the purpose of the anticipated group, which was to coordinate health equity efforts, develop one voice, and leverage resources. Their newly formed group agreed to draft a letter that would highlight specific language and recommendations for health disparities as part of comprehensive health care reform. The goal was to represent the priorities of as many organizations and coalitions as possible. They also decided to develop a "master list" of coalitions and organizations to better facilitate information dissemination and shared actions. Finally, they decided to send a sign-on letter to key committees requesting a hearing on health disparities to ensure congressional responsiveness. The letter, which was sent on April 16, 2009, was the first to come from this diverse group of advocates for disparate populations.

The result of this mobilization became formally known as the National Working Group on Health Disparities and Health Reform, a group of initially thirty-five organizations, associations, and coalitions that quickly grew and banded together to make health disparities elimination a priority during the health reform debates. The working group agreed to several overarching objectives to advance a health equity agenda in health reform, including (1) developing a robust advocacy strategy, (2) drafting model legislative language to incorporate in health reform proposals, (3) monitoring and analyzing any legislative proposals to ensure that they included health equity provisions, and (4) monitoring the implementation of these provisions.

Members of the working group convened weekly internal strategy meetings and external meetings with key congressional and administration officials. In the 111th Congress, Congresswoman Barbara Lee (D-CA) became chair of the forty-two-member Congressional Black Caucus, and several members were elevated to key positions leading the House Judiciary, Homeland Security, and Ways and Means Committees. Representative James Clyburn (D-SC) became the majority whip.

Their group worked closely not only with these champions for health reform but also with the Congressional Black Caucus Health Braintrust under the leadership of Congresswoman Christensen (D-VI); as well as with the Congressional Hispanic Caucus Health Care Task Force, under the leadership of Congresswoman Lucille Roybal-Allard; and the Congressional Asian Pacific American Caucus, under the leadership of Congressman Mike Honda (D-CA). The Tri-Caucus has proved to be a guardian of health equity and had long been a promoter and defender of policies in Congress intended to elevate the health of all communities.

The National Working Group also worked closely with the Congressional Native American Caucus, the White House, and key health policy-focused committees in Congress, including Energy and Commerce, Ways and Means, and Education and Labor. In one of the most contentious struggles over the chairmanship of the Energy and Commerce Committee, Congressman Henry Waxman, in a secret ballot vote in the Cannon Caucus Room, won the leadership position in a vote of 137–122. Essentially, Democrats in the House ratified an earlier decision by the Steering and Policy Committee to replace Congressman John Dingell Jr. (D-MI), the dean of the House of Representatives.

Waxman and his team had launched their challenge for this position the day after the November 2008 elections. Dingell and his team immediately launched a counteroffensive against Waxman and his supporters, but they ultimately lost to the Waxman machine, which had been lobbying behind the scenes to persuade other Democratic House members to support his bid and defy the seniority system that had long been in place. Some thought the eighty-two-year-old was too old and that Waxman, who was sixty-nine, would be better able to handle the expected intense and brutal negotiations over health reform. Nevertheless, Congressman Waxman, after winning the position, appointed Dingell chairman emeritus of the committee and allowed him to keep his office suite in the Capitol.

During the negotiations around health reform, both Waxman and his staff and Dingell and his staff worked cooperatively and closely on the health reform package in their committee. Although health equity proponents worked closely with Congressman Charles Rangel's staff on the Ways and Means Committee and Congressman George Miller's staff on the Education and Labor Committee, they spent more of their time working with both Waxman's and Dingell's staff to develop their bill before it was merged with the other two committees to become the Tri-Committee health reform bill. Waxman's team as well as Dingell's team worked closely with health equity proponents to understand and champion their priorities during internal committee negotiations over what provisions should be included in the bill. During their meetings with congressional members and staff, advocates emphasized that it had been almost ten years since President Bill Clinton signed into law the Minority Health and Health Disparities Research and Education Act of 2000, a critical but limited law on health disparities research and that the United States could not afford to wait another ten years to get more comprehensive legislation around health equity passed.

By the end of April 2009, their group had grown in the space of a month from 35 to more than 250 organizations, associations, and coalitions across the country. They were pleasantly surprised by the tremendous growth and interest in this group—word of mouth about their efforts was spreading like wildfire across the United States. People were calling and writing them, wanting to participate and to lend their voices to this cause. They represented diverse stakeholders, including consumers, racial and ethnic minorities, rural populations, people with disabilities, children, women, LGBTQ+ individuals, community health centers, hospitals and other health care entities, health professionals, insurers, and businesses. Their goal was to urge lawmakers and the Obama administration to ensure that any final comprehensive health reform legislation included provisions to address health inequities and to reduce and eliminate health care disparities. Like Obama, they, too, had developed an outline of issues they wanted included in health reform:

1. High-quality, affordable health care coverage must be available to everyone, particularly populations and communities that have traditionally suffered health disparities and barriers to coverage.
2. Health insurance coverage alone does not ensure access to health services. A full range of culturally and linguistically appropriate health care and public health services must be available in every community and accessible to all.

3. Every community must have the health workforce and infrastructure necessary to provide a full range of health care and public health services.
4. All efforts to reduce health disparities and barriers to quality health services require better data.
5. Recognition of diversity is critical to improving health care quality.

Growing Pains: More Progress, More Problems

During the expansion of the National Working Group, several key events occurred. On April 8, 2009, the president signed an executive order reemphasizing health reform as a key goal of his administration and establishing the White House Office of Health Reform and the Department of Health and Human Services Office of Health Reform. Both offices were ordered to coordinate closely with each other.[20] In the Senate, cooperation between the Senate Finance and HELP Committees on health reform increased. On April 20, 2009, Kennedy (chair of HELP) and Baucus (chair of Finance) sent a letter to Obama stating their mutual commitment to passing comprehensive health reform and marking up legislation in early June.

> Since their committees share jurisdiction over health care reform legislation in the Senate, they have jointly laid out an aggressive schedule to accomplish their goal. . . . Their intention is for that legislation to be very similar, and to reflect a shared approach to reform, so that the measures that their two committees report can be quickly merged into a single bill for consideration on the Senate floor.
>
> They have a moral duty to ensure that every American can get quality health care. They must act to contain the growth of health care costs to ensure their economic stability; to help American businesses deal with the health care challenge; and to make sure that they are getting their money's worth. With your continued leadership and commitment, and working together, they remain certain that their goal of enacting comprehensive health care reform can be accomplished with the urgency that the American people rightly demand.[21]

In previous attempts to pass health reform legislation, these committees had competed against each other instead of working together on a bill. This demonstration of unity signaled to health law and policy experts that health reform stood a serious chance of passing. The following day, Baucus and Grassley held the first of three roundtables, bringing together health policy and industry experts to discuss the development of health care reform legislation.

One week after its joint letter to the president and its first roundtable, the Senate Finance Committee on April 28, 2009, released detailed policy options for reforming America's health care delivery system, which was the first of three sets of policy options released publicly for members of Congress and the public to review.[22] This was in keeping with the committee's track record of producing resources aimed at influencing the health reform agenda.

After the first set of policy options was released, the National Working Group attempted to meet with the Senate Finance Committee to discuss the inclusion of provisions aimed at increasing access to quality health care and public health services, research on health disparities, cultural competence, and more robust and accurate data collection and reporting. At first, the committee ignored their requests to meet. Fact sheets, issue briefs, and other materials they created to inform committee members were never acknowledged, nor was any language the working group offered for inclusion in the first policy paper accepted. They became troubled that the leading committee on health reform in the Senate seemingly failed to appreciate the seriousness of their issues. Members of the National Working Group then reached out to American Indian tribes in Montana since Baucus represented that state and was the chair of the Senate Finance Committee and discussed their concerns. Members of the Montana American Indian community made sure to voice their disapproval to the committee for failing to meet with members of the National Working Group. After this occurred, members of their group were finally given an audience with senior staff on the Finance Committee.

From the Senate HELP Committee, they experienced quite a different reception. Kennedy, who had long been a champion for addressing health disparities and had previously worked with Senator Bill Frist (R-TN) to develop legislation tackling this issue, agreed that provisions directly addressing the problem should be included in any health reform proposal. His staff worked diligently to negotiate these priorities in committee along with senior staff from other Senate offices. When seeking individual champions on the two committees of jurisdiction in the Senate over health policy, advocates encountered both supportive and unsupportive staff, and senators who either did not see the relevance of including their provisions or thought them too controversial. Many senators and their staff deemed these health equity provisions deal killers for the larger health reform bill, despite the advocates' best efforts to demonstrate how these priorities had long enjoyed bipartisan support.

One Democratic senator's staff, for instance, employed a tactic designed to keep health equity advocates thinking they stood a chance to have their issue addressed: the staff person, knowing full well no Republican was on board with health reform at that point, told advocates they would consider their legislative priorities if they secured a Republican co-sponsor. Early on, when they knew Republicans were not going to support any health reform package, they decided to focus their attention on Democrats who were proponents of health reform and launch an educational and advocacy campaign to advance health equity. Senators Harry Reid (D-NV), Ben Cardin (D-MD), Barbara Mikulski (D-MD), Tom Harkin (D-IA), Richard Durbin (D-IL), Daniel Inouye (D-HI), Daniel Akaka (D-HI), and Roland Burris (D-IL) became their primary champions in the Senate.[23]

While there was increasing unity among old congressional competitors, members within the group were beginning to express dissatisfaction with the National Working Group, concerned that their priorities were not being addressed. Advocates from the disability community began to push back against other members of the National Working Group, complaining about insufficient language relating to the disability community in group letters. The LGBTQ+ community also was equally upset about materials not explicitly mentioning their issues. Likewise, advocates from the racial and ethnic minority community voiced concern about losing ground since health disparities had long been focused on them. All of these communities were informed that the larger group letters that they created were purposely designed to address health disparities broadly and that it was up to each group to speak out for its respective population. Moreover, the National Working Group reminded them that they had not yet received any specific language, except on one or two occasions, to include in their material. Eventually, these disagreements faded and the diverse stakeholders continued to collaborate to push for health equity.

Seeing Government as a Partner, Not as an Adversary

While communicating with congressional health reform champions, members of the National Working Group were also corresponding with the White House to prioritize health equity in the negotiations. The Department of Health and Human Services and the White House Office of Health Reform expressed interest in mid-April in scheduling a meeting or an event around health disparities. They remained persistent in pushing this issue, even as White House staffers were moving slowly in scheduling the meeting. The National Working Group continued forward with their efforts and on April 22 held their second meeting, which was attended by Senate HELP Committee staff. After the meeting, the group sent out an email summarizing their agenda and announcing their next meeting.

On April 29, 2009, the White House Office of National AIDS Policy convened a meeting with a select group of health reform stakeholders, which some members of the National Working Group attended. One individual, who had helped to organize the National Working Group, worked tirelessly to secure this meeting. The objectives of the meeting were to (1) highlight the challenges of HIV/AIDS prevention, treatment, and care and the less than optimal response at the federal level; (2) identify the HIV/AIDS community's needs and highlight the responses that had been pursued; (3) facilitate involvement of the underserved community (e.g., regular meetings, conversations) in the development of a national AIDS strategy; (4) frame the issue as an example of a health disparity for underserved communities; and (5) encourage the inclusion of this and other health disparities in the overall national health reform conversation. Although they were pleased that the issue of health disparities was included in this discussion, members of the National Working Group took the opportunity to ask for a follow-up meeting with the White House Office of Health Reform dedicated to the issue of health disparities, specifically the inclusion of health equity in health reform.

The following day, the third meeting of the National Working Group took place. They finalized the second letter to send to key members of Congress and administration officials requesting the inclusion of health disparities as a part of comprehensive health reform. They continued developing a master list of coalitions, groups, and organizations committed to this cause. The group coordinated congressional visits and began developing talking points on health disparities for these visits. The framework for the talking points would follow along the lines of categories delineated by the Senate HELP Committee: (1) coverage, (2) access, (3) quality, (4) service delivery, and (5) data collection. They also discussed developing a website that would highlight all submitted recommendations, principles, and documents on health disparities as an additional tool for congressional staff to incorporate stakeholder recommendations when crafting health reform legislation.

On May 11, 2009, the Senate Finance Committee published its second set of policy options, focused on expanding health care coverage. These options included an entire section on health equity, titled "Options to Address Health Disparities." This section was a direct result of the National Working Group's persistent advocacy efforts—their recommendations were instrumental in the final product. The proposed options would expand data collection measures; require health care quality data to be published by race, ethnicity, and gender; expand translation services for Medicaid beneficiaries; and allow states to waive the five-year waiting period for Medicaid coverage. In the announcement, Baucus, the Senate Finance Committee chair, made an economic argument: "Expanding health care coverage is not just a moral imperative—it's an economic necessity. . . . These policy options propose a uniquely American approach to provide affordable, quality coverage to all Americans through a mix of public and private solutions, and drive down health care costs for every American."[24]

Gaining and Sustaining the Government's Support for Health Equity: What's the Government Investment Value?

May 2009 was a particularly busy month for the National Working Group. It was a period of intense activity, and they worked long, grueling hours strategizing, responding to congressional requests, drafting model legislative language, and writing letters and messages. They had to be careful with their language at all times to avoid the risk of alienating members from any of the groups represented in the National Working Group. Their second letter, supporting the Senate Finance Committee's inclusion of health equity options and seeking to ensure that other committees also included health disparities provisions, was finalized and sent to members of Congress and the White House on May 6, 2009.

They created a group LISTSERV to help with scheduling congressional meetings and sharing information between National Working Group members. They also created advocacy packets containing information on various health equity issues and drafted and vetted a cover letter to include with them. Finally, they created and unveiled a website to house materials developed by group members, which served as a comprehensive database of information on health disparities accessible to policy makers.

The National Working Group continued on, and at their next meeting, they hammered out their talking points, organized visits to Capitol

Hill, and considered organizing a congressional briefing on health disparities. The Congressional Black Caucus was alarmed by the inadequate attention focused on racial and ethnic health disparities and started to pressure the Obama administration to increase its support for this issue in the health reform bills. Members of the CBC were particularly upset that the president had not included reference to addressing disparities in health care in his June 2, 2009, letter to Kennedy and Baucus.[25] Obama's letter made the case for tackling health reform because of the escalating health care costs that were bankrupting families and straining health care delivery. He argued the need for various delivery system and payment system reforms, such as accountable care organizations, and for cuts to Medicare and Medicaid spending, and he expressed interest in their ideas around shared responsibility, but he did not mention the impact of health disparities and their tremendous economic burden on their nation.

Three days after the president sent his letter to the chairs of the two Senate committees that had jurisdiction over health policy issues, the CBC issued an advisory alerting the media of a health equity news conference they planned to convene June 9 at 10 a.m. and sent a letter to the president firmly urging him to ensure that health equity remained an integral component of health reform. The caucus was troubled that some in the administration seemed to believe that health insurance coverage alone would meaningfully tackle racial and ethnic health disparities. It wanted assurance that the president kept his promise about addressing health disparities in health reform legislation that he made during his first health reform town hall at the White House. In the CBC letter, Barbara Lee, Donna Christensen, and Danny K. Davis strongly urged the president "to ensure that efforts to reform the nation's health care system integrate aggressive solutions to the nation's current plight with pervasive health disparities" and asserted that health reform efforts should "include provisions that address the root causes of all health inequities." They also stated, "We, like you, share a keen interest in ensuring that as we work together to reform the nation's health care system, that we do so in a manner that truly transforms it into one that serves all Americans appropriately, consistently, and equitably, regardless of their racial and ethnic background, gender, geography, language preference, or sexual orientation."[26]

As a result of the efforts by the Tri-Caucus, especially the CBC, and the National Working Group, health equity advocates achieved a major breakthrough in June when the White House agreed to convene a stakeholder meeting on health disparities and health reform, confirming that these concerns were indeed being treated as a priority. On June 9, several health disparities experts, most of them members of the National Working Group, met with Secretary Kathleen Sebelius; Nancy-Ann DeParle, director of the White House Office of Health Reform; and Tina Tchen, chief of staff to First Lady Michelle Obama. Participants in this meeting thought it was fitting that the meeting was held in the Indian Treaty Room at the Eisenhower Executive Office Building because it gave them a sense that the White House deemed this issue important enough to host it in a room that has long been associated with major announcements or events in the nation's history. Participants were given approximately two minutes each to discuss their priorities for health reform and how the health reform proposals could address health disparities.

During the meeting, advocates tried to reinforce their health equity priorities: that high-quality, affordable health care coverage must be available to everyone, particularly underresourced communities, and that every community must have the health workforce and infrastructure necessary to provide a full range of health care and public health services. They also emphasized that governments and health providers must be required to support the collection and accurate reporting of standardized demographic data on patients and the community and be provided the resources to do so. They recognized that, without that data, the disparities in health care among these marginalized groups could not be accurately tracked. In addition, during the meeting, the Department of Health and Human Services released a report on health disparities titled *Health Disparities: A Case for Closing the Gap.*

June 9, 2009, was certainly a busy day for health equity advocates. In addition to the White House's stakeholder meeting on health disparities and health reform, the Senate HELP Committee released a draft health reform bill that included health equity provisions—the Affordable Health Choices Act—and the Congressional Tri-Caucus released a draft of its comprehensive health equity bill—the Health Equity and Accountability Act of 2009—which was officially introduced on June 26, 2006, by Congresswoman Christensen on the Energy and Commerce Committee.

On June 10, 2010, the Ways and Means Subcommittee on Health, under the leadership of Chair Fortney Pete Stark (D-CA) and ranking member Dave Camp (R-MI), held the first-ever hearing focused solely on health disparities for that committee, titled *Addressing Disparities in Health*

and Healthcare: Issues of Reform. Both Stark and Camp recognized that, although health insurance coverage would put "a dent in addressing disparities," insurance coverage alone would not resolve the crisis.[27] For months,
health equity champions had been pushing congressional leaders on both
sides of the aisle to convene a hearing on this critical issue and were thrilled
that once again their voices had been heard and their request for a hearing
was granted.

Due in part to the incredible advocacy of Congressman Xavier Becerra
(D-CA) and Congresswoman Stephanie Tubbs Jones (D-OH), the subcommittee decided to dedicate one hearing to addressing this issue and fleshing out priorities. Witnesses included three Tri-Caucus members: Congress-
women Donna M. Christensen, Hilda L. Solis, and Madeleine Z. Bordallo
(D-Guam). In addition, representatives from several organizations, including the Kaiser Family Foundation, the National Medical Association, the
Asian & Pacific Islander American Health Forum, and the American Enterprise Institute were also invited to give testimony. Other groups that
provided written submissions included the American Dental Education Association, America's Health Insurance Plans, American College of Physicians, American Hospital Association, National Council of Urban Indian
Health, the National Black Nurses Association, and the Special Olympics
International.

During what was arguably the busiest week for health equity advocacy during the entire negotiations around health reform in 2009, one
other noteworthy event was convened. On Friday, June 12, 2009, the US
Commission on Civil Rights, which is an independent, bipartisan agency
established by Congress in 1957 charged with monitoring federal civil
rights enforcement, held a public briefing to examine the reasons for persistent gaps between the health status of minorities and nonminorities in
the United States.[28] Several health equity experts presented testimony
highlighting the need to increase the diversity and cultural competence
of the health professions workforce; address data collection gaps and
challenges especially for subpopulation groups; address the multifactorial
causes of disparities and the interplay among socioeconomic, environmental, individual, and personal factors as well as other social determinants of health; improve the quality of care and address the need for culturally and linguistically appropriate care; and address unconscious bias
in health care.

Dr. Sally Satel, a scholar with the American Enterprise Institute, also
testified that there were indeed disparities among minorities, but she

argued that the causes of these disparities were debatable. She sought to discredit the National Academy of Medicine's *Unequal Treatment* report, which comprehensively highlighted troubling disparities in the US health care system by outlining what she perceived to be some of its methodological problems. She concluded that "the elimination of health differentials is not feasible because they cannot eliminate the disparities, the social disparities, many of which take their most profound toll in terms of the habits of mind and view of the future. Such an agenda clearly transcends the work of public health and is best left to politicians, voters and social welfare experts."[29]

Throughout the negotiations, they continued to hear others raise the points she had made, particularly that it is impossible to eliminate disparities because approximately 50 percent of the disparities in health result from social and physical determinants of health that are out of any provider's control. Some argued that providers have significant control over the 20 percent of input related to clinical care and shared control over 30 percent related to health behaviors, but when it comes to socioeconomic factors (40 percent) and physical environment (10 percent), hospitals and physicians have limited control and capabilities.

Health equity advocates pushed back, however, and argued that many of these social and physical determinants of health transpired because of past practices and promulgation of policies that could be addressed through meaningful collaboration with community stakeholders and leaders.[30] Which is why, although Satel failed to appreciate the scope, depth, and complexity of health inequities by dismissing the work that public health plays in systematically addressing this multifactorial problem, she raised an important point about the role that politicians and voters play in tackling this issue. Improving the social determinants of health alone will not ensure health equity. Health equity proponents must also tackle the political determinants of health, which are, arguably, the determinants of the determinants, to effect the changes necessary to achieve this goal.

Two weeks after the White House's stakeholder meeting, health equity advocates mobilized and held a rally on the evening of June 24, 2009—Lighting the Night: Healthcare Equality '09—at Freedom Plaza in Washington, DC. This rally, which was sponsored by the Service Employees International Union Healthcare Equality Project, brought hundreds of people from across the country to demand that health reform truly work for everyone. Rally participants believed that health care had to go beyond simply expanding coverage to all uninsured Americans; it had to put us on a path toward health care equality. Participants also believed that all people, no matter the color of their skin, deserve affordable, accessible health care of the highest quality. The venue provided an opportunity for advocates to speak out to demand health care equity, enjoy cultural foods and live entertainment, culminate the evening with a candlelight vigil to symbolize the power of the health equity movement, and urge their members of Congress to fight for equitable reform. During the event, Congresswoman Roybal-Allard, chair of the Congressional Hispanic Caucus Health Care Task Force, joined the rally and urged health equity champions to continue their fight for health equity. She stated, "I stand with you in our shared commitment to achieve a nation free of health disparities, with quality health outcomes for all, regardless of ethnic, racial or cultural background. For we all know that the only way to improve the health of ALL Americans is to enhance the health of EVERY American."[31]

In July 2009, the National Working Group conducted a comprehensive strategic advocacy campaign, which entailed holding meetings with key officials over several weeks to underscore the impact of health disparities on the population. They argued that including health equity provisions in health reform legislation would result in greatly improved health and thousands of lives saved. The National Working Group at this time also sent a third letter to Congress urging support for the inclusion of the comprehensive Health Equity and Accountability Act of 2009 in health reform proposals. It had been introduced in every Congress since 2003 by the Tri-Caucus, which included the Congressional Black Caucus, the Congressional Hispanic Caucus, and the Congressional Asian Pacific American Caucus.

Never Underestimate the Opposition: Moving Through the Headwinds

At this time, as health reform bills in the House were taking shape and negative ads against health reform efforts in Congress were sweeping the country, several congressional members and staff who were supportive of health equity and passing comprehensive health reform legislation contacted advocates, urging them to more publicly demonstrate their support for health reform. Lawmakers expressed concern that they were hearing only from individuals who opposed the legislation, so a strong show of support for health reform legislation would be needed to

Advocacy Action Steps

Injustice must be rooted out by strong, persistent and determined action.—Dr. Martin Luther King Jr.

Once health equity advocates formed the National Working Group on Health Disparities and Health Reform, which ultimately included more than three hundred national organizations, associations, and coalitions committed to health equity, they immediately went to work developing and implementing a flexible advocacy strategy around communications and media, grassroots, and outreach to Congress and the Obama administration, including Tri-Caucus members. This flexible approach allowed group members to sequentially and simultaneously develop and implement certain components of the advocacy strategy depending on various existing and emerging factors.

The first step in organizing the group and ensuring better facilitation of information dissemination among group members internally was to create a master list of all organizations, associations, and coalitions committed to the inclusion of health equity provisions in health reform. Each organization was urged to specify its areas of expertise around health disparities in regard to quality improvement, behavioral health, prevention and public health, research, and workforce development.

Their second action step was to identify and recruit external champions of health equity in Congress and the administration, as well as organizations that had not yet joined the group, including health care, behavioral health, and public health experts in Washington, DC, and around the country. The intent of this action step was to get health equity included in the larger health reform discussions that were taking place around prevention and wellness, quality improvement, workforce development, insurance expansion, and comparative effectiveness research.

The third action step of the advocacy strategy was to collect and share stories about different populations that were experiencing inequities in health care and public health. One such story was that of Esmin Green, who died at a hospital after being ignored by guards and medical staff. Advocates used this story as a wake-up call to show that health care disparities are real and can have tragic consequences. The story also served to highlight the lack of compassion toward individuals with mental health problems and the need for more culturally competent health professionals. Stories such as Esmin Green's were effective in putting a face to the somewhat abstract problem of health disparities.

The fourth action step included the initiation of a postcard and letter campaign to congressional leadership explaining the importance of addressing health disparities and urging them to support the inclusion of health equity provisions in health reform legislation.

Advocacy Action Steps

The fifth action step involved developing health equity principles, talking points, legislative outlines, and legislative language to share with the key congressional committees charged with drafting the health reform bill.

The sixth action step by the group involved holding congressional meetings and briefings to educate members of Congress about this critical issue and to serve as a reminder that health equity advocates were persistent and adamant about the inclusion of robust provisions in health reform to address health disparities.

Overall, the convening of the National Working Group on Health Disparities and Health Reform resulted in enhanced cooperation, as well as efficient and more targeted use of resources to overcome challenges and leverage opportunities. It led to the creation and execution of a more effective strategy to inform members of Congress and the Obama administration about health disparities, their impact on the health status and care of vulnerable populations, and the cost burden to the United States.

secure enough votes for passage. Emotions were high, Democrats were on edge, and many were politically fatigued because of the ambitious legislative undertaking they had endured since the beginning of the year—from tackling the financial bailout of major banking institutions to stimulating the economy out of the Great Recession to climate change and other major bills.

The concern about the show of support from health reform champions arose in part from the increasing complexity of the health reform bills and the emergence earlier in the year of the Tea Party, a conservative populist movement characterized by ire against the federal government and what they perceived as excessive taxation. Many Democratic lawmakers were concerned about how comprehensive the bill had become, and "few in the caucus of 256 House Democrats [understood] the emerging 1,000-page bill."[32] To rectify this internal problem, House Democratic leaders organized several briefings during various stages of the bills to keep members informed about what was taking place in the committees that were working on the bills.

While congressional leaders addressed concerns internally in their caucus, they relied on external groups to help them more broadly inform the public about the health reform proposals and stave off rampant misinformation that was engulfing districts across the United States. Tea Party members were virulently opposed to health reform and expended much effort in protesting it. Their protests were spurred on by onetime vice presidential nominee Sarah Palin, who claimed that the health reform legislation would create "death panels" of government employees who would decide who could receive care. Palin was at the time referring to a provision in the early bill that would allow Medicare to cover end-of-life counseling. The furor from Palin's claim led to this provision's removal from the legislation. Palin later claimed that she was referring to the Independent Payment Advisory Board, a committee tasked with controlling the rate of Medicare spending.[33] Though inaccurate, Palin's notion of "death panels" took hold among the public, fueling Tea Party resistance.

The leaders of the National Working Group therefore reached out to their members, mobilizing their grassroots to send a clear message to Congress that they supported this vital legislation. With the rise of the Tea Party movement, health reform champions were faced with a new, bold, and uncooperative force opposing the passage of any health reform bill. Members of the Tea Party fanned the flames of resentment, amplified the opposition's voice, and retaliated with the fiercest measures. None-theless, during this time of increased opposition, congressional health reformers demonstrated indefatigable courage and resolve, continuing to push for comprehensive health reform despite the tide of external pressures and the unrelenting campaign to dismantle any health reform package that had advanced in the House and Senate. Like previous Congresses, the 111th Congress found itself at a critical juncture in the nation's history, one that presented both an opportunity and a challenge: whether to stand up for what is right even though it may not be popular at the time.

In a surprising turnaround, the American Medical Association on July 16, 2009, boldly announced its support for the House's health reform bill. The AMA spoke favorably of the bill's provisions that were "key to effective, comprehensive health reform," including providing choice of plans through health insurance exchanges, ending coverage denials based on preexisting conditions, and providing additional funding for primary care services. In an interview on the subject the following week, their president explained the organization's decision to support health care reform: "The AMA is clearly committed to health reform this year. We believe the status quo is unacceptable. We want to make sure patients have access to a healthcare system that has affordable health insurance coverage for everybody. As we took a look at those principles and the bill that was being proposed, we knew that our endorsement would be helpful to keep the legislative process moving forward."[34] Given the history of the advocacy around health reform and that the AMA had in the past been its fiercest opponent, this reversal from one of the most powerful associations in health care was a major boon for the prospects of enacting health reform.

Shaping the Policy: Reform for All, Not Reform for Some!

Despite making strides with the White House and lawmakers, the secondary treatment of the issue of health disparities was still evident during negotiations. Nevertheless, the working group, finding strength in numbers and harnessing the power of collaboration, pushed forward, arguing that it was imperative for policy makers to acknowledge the severity of the problems and enact health reforms to curb them. Health equity advocates frequently and consistently argued that eliminating disparities should be a key component of health reform since it would improve health status, save lives, and increase longevity and quality of life for the nation's most vulnerable populations. The National Working Group's tag line became *Health reform should be reform for all, not reform for some!*

The National Working Group on Health Disparities and Health Reform, which by August 2009 had grown to include well over three hundred national organizations, associations, and coalitions, tirelessly advocated for health equity provisions, which endured multiple attacks from those opposed to health equity or those simply ignorant about these issues. For several months, the working group argued that including health equity provisions in health reform would result in greatly improved health and thousands of lives saved. They thought this moral argument would be sufficient to ensure the inclusion of health equity provisions, and it seemed to resonate with many members of Congress and their staff. But then the focus shifted to costs and cost savings. The Congressional Budget Office analysis estimated that the provisions of the health reform bills would cost more than $1 trillion, so House and Senate health reformers felt tremendous pressure to reduce the estimated costs of their bills.[35] The White House also felt pressure to counter arguments that health reform was unaffordable and that the country could not pass a health reform package costing more than $1 trillion because it would increase the national deficit.

The working group had to react and reframe their message to accommodate this new focus and demonstrate the cost burden of health and health care disparities on the country. That was easier said than done. Up to this point, group members had tried their best to engage in proactive advocacy, but the shift in focus by policy makers forced advocates to employ a reactive advocacy strategy to accommodate this new shift and to ensure the continued relevance of health equity provisions in the larger debate on health reform. When congressional staff requested information on the costs of health disparities and the cost savings that would be realized by reducing these disparities, the National Working Group was able to share only two very small studies focusing on Colorado and California.

Fortunately, the Joint Center for Political and Economic Studies released a groundbreaking report by Johns Hopkins University and George Washington University researchers Drs. Thomas A. LaVeist, Darrell J. Gaskin, and Patrick Richard on the costs of health disparities in the United States, which put things into perspective.[36] The numbers were more frightening than many thought. But at least now, health equity advocates were able to convince congressional staff that they could not afford to ignore health disparities in health reform. Their working group ardently voiced support for the notion that cost savings would be realized not only by improving the health of populations and communities that experience health disparities and barriers to health care and public health services but also by reducing the costs resulting from the disproportionate burden of disease faced by these populations. Unfortunately, demonstrating the cost savings that would accrue to the United States if it reduced and eliminated health disparities was not enough to convince policy makers for long, because the focus for health reform shifted once again. Policy makers moved away from calling health reform "comprehensive health reform" to "health insurance reform" once opposition to the bill started to intensify. On August 8, 2009, in his weekly address, the president for the first time referred to health reform as "health insurance reform."[37]

At first, many members of the National Working Group thought this was a smart shift—vilifying the insurance companies. But then they became concerned when many government officials started taking a narrow approach to health reform, primarily discussing health insurance coverage provisions and barely mentioning the other provisions around quality, prevention, and health workforce. Health equity advocates argued that health insurance coverage was crucial, but addressing it alone would not necessarily equate to access and access would not necessarily equate to quality services, treatment, and better outcomes. The group further argued that they envisioned health reform legislation that ensured equity and accountability, provided individuals with the ability to access comprehensive and culturally and linguistically appropriate health care and public health services, and achieved health outcomes consistent with the rest of the population.

From "Comprehensive Health Reform" to "Health Insurance Reform"

■ On March 5, 2009, during a special forum on health reform, President Barack Obama declared, "Their goal will be to enact *comprehensive health reform* by the end of this year."[1]

■ On April 20, 2009, Senator Edward Kennedy (chair of Senate HELP Committee) and Senator Max Baucus (chair of Senate Finance Committee) sent a letter to President Obama affirming their mutual commitment to passing "*comprehensive health reform*" and marking up legislation in early June.[2]

■ On May 13, 2009, the president wrote in his first email newsletter, "The Vice President and I just met with leaders from the House of Representatives and received their commitment to pass a '*comprehensive health care reform*' bill by July 31."[3]

■ On June 2, 2009, President Obama sent a lengthy letter to both Senators Kennedy and Baucus, where it was clear the administration had nixed "comprehensive" when describing health care reform. He commended them for "the hard work your Committees are doing on *health care reform*" and stated "*health care reform* is not a luxury." He went on to say, "They simply cannot afford to postpone *health care reform* any longer" and "*health care reform* must not add to their deficits over the next 10 years." He then concluded by mentioning "health care reform" three more times, including that he was "committed to working with the Congress to fully offset the cost of *health care reform*," that there was "a valuable tool to help achieve *health care reform*," and that he "look[ed] forward to working with [them] so that the Congress can complete *health care reform* by October."[4] In all, the president mentioned health care reform seven times in his letter. This was a noticeable change in strategy—moving from "comprehensive health reform" to "health care reform," which occurred at the height of the Tea Party's emergence, when congressional staffers were asking health reform proponents to make their voices heard more.

■ On June 15, 2009, President Obama during his speech at the annual conference of the AMA, continued referencing "health care reform" and moved away from using "comprehensive health reform," except one time when he referred to "comprehensive reform." He said, "After all, Presidents have called for *health care reform* for nearly a century." Later on he mentioned, "They know the moment is right for *health care reform*" and "*health care reform* should be guided by a simple principle: Fix what's broken and build on what works." He also emphasized, "*Health care reform* must be, and will be, deficit-neutral in the next decade," and "the best thing for their charities is the stronger economy that they will build with *health care reform*." And he stated, "They've put $950 billion on the table, taking us almost all the way to covering the full cost of *health care reform*," and "I look forward to working with Congress to make up the difference so that *health care reform* is fully paid for."[5]

■ On July 17, 2009, President Obama made remarks pledging to get *health care reform* done that year. Remarks did not include the term "comprehensive."[6]

■ On August 8, 2009, President Obama in his weekly address stated, "They must lay a new foundation for future growth and prosperity, and a key pillar of a new foundation is *health insurance reform*—reform that they are now closer to achieving than ever before."[7]

■ On October 29, 2009, Speaker Nancy Pelosi and the House Democratic Caucus held an event at the Capitol on *health insurance reform*.

■ On November 21, 2009, Senator Patrick Leahy, speaking on the floor of the Senate stated, "Decision time is near on *health insurance reform*."[8]

■ On December 24, 2009, President Obama, after the vote in the Senate, made remarks that included reference to health insurance reform three times. First, he remarked, "In a historic vote that took place this morning members of the Senate joined their colleagues in the House of Representatives to pass a landmark *health insurance reform package*." Second, he asserted, "They are now finally poised to deliver on the promise of real, meaningful *health insurance reform*." Third he stated, "They are now incredibly close to making *health insurance reform* a reality in this country."[9]

■ On March 21, 2010, Speaker Pelosi spoke on the House floor before the vote on the Patient Protection and Affordable Care Act: "Today, they have the opportunity to complete the great unfinished business of their society and pass *health insurance reform* for all Americans that is a right and not a privilege."[10]

Notes

1. Obama, "Remarks by the President at the Opening of the White House Forum on Health Reform" (emphasis added).
2. Newton-Small, "And. Here. They. Go" (emphasis added).
3. Lee, "Health Reform" (emphasis added).
4. Lee, "The President Spells Out His Vision on Health Care Reform" (emphasis added).
5. Obama, "Remarks by the President to the Annual Conference of the American Medical Association" (emphasis added).
6. Brandon, "President on Health Care" (emphasis added).
7. Obama, "President Obama Calls Health Insurance Reform Key to Stronger Economy and Improvement on Status Quo" (emphasis added).
8. Cong. Rec. S11907–S11967 (November 21, 2009, emphasis added).
9. Obama, "Remarks by the President on Senate Passage of Health Insurance Reform" (emphasis added).
10. Pelosi, "Today, They Have the Opportunity to Complete the Great Unfinished Business of Their Society and Pass Health Insurance Reform for All Americans" (emphasis added).

5
Winning the Game That Never Ends
Success Means Continuous Employment of the Political Determinants of Health

We have the oldest written constitution still in force in the world, and it starts out with three words, "We, the people."—*Ruth Bader Ginsburg, US Supreme Court Justice*

Balancing the Dialogue: Untangling Legitimate Concerns from Plain Obstruction

During August 2009, the period that Congress typically takes off to visit constituents, the Tea Party movement executed a strategy to target town halls that were convened by Democrats. These town halls resulted in heated exchanges between the member of Congress and the audience. House Speaker Nancy Pelosi, echoing the sentiments of many in her caucus, declared that "the town hall meetings were really an orchestration. What is out there's where people who want to stop a progress, exploit and hijack the good intentions of people who have legitimate concerns. So you have to be able to differentiate among those who are obstructionists and those who have real concerns."[1] Health reform supporters did their best to mobilize their base and ensure that the dialogue was balanced, but they were no match for the opposition groups who heckled lawmakers and effectively spread propaganda.

On August 25, 2009, Senator Edward Kennedy, the great champion for health reform, passed away, just one month after his Senate Health, Education, Labor and Pensions Committee passed the Affordable Health Choices Act. So strong was Senator Kennedy's passion for health reform that, in 2008, he ignored his doctors' advice and gave a speech at the Democratic National Convention in Denver about health care reform. In May 2009, he repeated his feelings in a letter to President Obama, which his wife, Vicki, delivered after his passing. "You will be the president who at long last signs into law the health care reform that is the great unfinished business of our society," Kennedy wrote. "For me, this cause stretched across decades; it has been disappointed, but never finally defeated. It was the cause of my life."[2] A few weeks later Obama gave remarks to a joint session of Congress on health care, supporting the ongoing negotiations in Congress, and reemphasizing his commitment to reform. Obama spoke about Kennedy during his remarks:

> Now, I have no interest in putting insurance companies out of business. They provide a legitimate service, and employ a lot of our friends and neighbors. I just want to hold them accountable. (Applause.) And the insurance reforms that I've already mentioned would do just that. But an additional step we can take to keep insurance companies honest is by making a not-for-profit public option available in the insurance exchange. (Applause.) Now, let me be clear. Let me be clear. It would only be an option for those who don't have insurance. No one would be forced to choose it, and it would not impact those of you who already have insurance. In fact, based on Congressional Budget Office estimates, we believe that less than 5 percent of Americans would sign up.
>
> Despite all this, the insurance companies and their allies don't like this idea. They argue that these private companies can't fairly compete with the government. And they'd be right if taxpayers were subsidizing this public insurance option. But they won't be. I've insisted that like any private insurance company, the public insurance option would have to be self-sufficient and rely on the premiums it collects. But by avoiding some of the overhead that gets eaten up at private companies by profits and excessive administrative costs and executive salaries, it could provide a good deal for consumers, and would also keep pressure on private insurers to keep their policies affordable and treat their customers better, the same way public colleges and universities provide additional choice and competition to students without in any way inhibiting a vibrant system of private colleges and universities. (Applause.)
>
> Now, it is—it's worth noting that a strong majority of Americans still favor a public insurance option of the sort I've proposed tonight. But its impact shouldn't be exaggerated—by the left or the right or the media. It is only one part of my plan, and shouldn't be used as a handy excuse for the usual Washington ideological battles. To my progressive friends, I would remind you that for decades, the driving idea behind reform has been to end insurance company abuses and make coverage available for those without it. (Applause.) The public option—the public option is only a means to that end—and we should remain open to other ideas that accomplish our ultimate goal. And to my Republican friends, I say that rather than making wild claims

about a government takeover of health care, we should work together to address any legitimate concerns you may have. (Applause.)

I received one of those letters a few days ago. It was from our beloved friend and colleague, Ted Kennedy. He had written it back in May, shortly after he was told that his illness was terminal. He asked that it be delivered upon his death.

In it, he spoke about what a happy time his last months were, thanks to the love and support of family and friends, his wife, Vicki, his amazing children, who are all here tonight. And he expressed confidence that this would be the year that health care reform—"that great unfinished business of our society," he called it—would finally pass. He repeated the truth that health care is decisive for our future prosperity, but he also reminded me that "it concerns more than material things." "What we face," he wrote, "is above all a moral issue; at stake are not just the details of policy, but fundamental principles of social justice and the character of our country."

I've thought about that phrase quite a bit in recent days—the character of our country. One of the unique and wonderful things about America has always been our self-reliance, our rugged individualism, our fierce defense of freedom and our healthy skepticism of government. And figuring out the appropriate size and role of government has always been a source of rigorous and, yes, sometimes angry debate. That's our history.[3]

Both Kennedy and Obama highlighted the moral imperative of passing health reform and its fundamental role in elevating social justice during the midpoint of the negotiations after having focused on economic and national security arguments. At this point, policy makers and health equity proponents had made all four major arguments in support of health reform: moral, outcomes, economic, and national security.

When Kennedy lost his battle with cancer on August 25, 2009, there was a sense that advocates had lost a great leader, one who through experience had the wherewithal to finally help usher in the successful passage of health reform. Perhaps realizing the impact his death could have on passing the health reform legislation if Democrats lost their sixty-vote majority in the Senate, Kennedy had earlier requested that the Massachusetts legislature enact a law allowing the governor to appoint a temporary replacement until a special election could be held. The legislature did so, and Massachusetts governor Deval Patrick appointed Paul G. Kirk Jr., a former aide of the late senator, to fill his seat until a special election on January 19, 2010.

However, under the Massachusetts Constitution, unless a law is an emergency or declared so by the governor, it cannot take effect earlier than ninety days after it is passed. Patrick declared that Kirk's appointment was indeed an emergency. However, while Kirk enjoyed tremendous support from Obama and other Democratic leaders, Republicans were not especially pleased with his selection. They argued that it was unconstitutional for the governor to make an emergency declaration in this case and set out to get an injunction to prevent the appointment from taking effect. Their efforts were not successful, and Kirk's appointment remained.

After fighting to make sure that other health equity provisions remained a priority during this shift to "health insurance reform," advocates endured additional battles and had to make sure that they remained diligent in their advocacy in order to keep these provisions intact. On September 2, 2009, the advocates were contacted by White House officials warning them that several of their health equity provisions were slated for the chopping block. The advocates were surprised to hear this and conveyed to White House officials their concerns. Then, the following morning, the *New York Times* published an article titled "Obama Aides Aim to Scale Back Health Bills," which detailed plans by some officials to eliminate provisions in health reform proposals around data collection and school-based health clinics.[4] The White House raised a cost argument, stating that it would raise the cost of the bill if they were to remain. However, health equity proponents pushed back stating these provisions would, in the long run, actually reduce the costs to the government and ultimately the taxpayers. They were disappointed but determined to keep pushing back against any attempts to repeal their critical provisions.

The Congressional Black Caucus was also deeply concerned about the possibility that the public option and key health equity provisions could be stricken. The next day, on September 3, 2009, the CBC struck back by declaring its strong opposition to any attempts to cut the myriad of health disparity elimination provisions. Anticipating the president's address before a joint session of Congress in one week, the CBC used its letter to highlight its key priorities as health reform continued to move forward: (1) shifting the focus away from the substance of the bill to the cost of the bill would be ineffective, (2) the need for a strong public option, (3) commitment from the White House to use health reform to achieve health equity, (4) inclusion of provisions to ensure equity and parity for individuals in the US territories, and (5) the use of savings from the prevention and public health provisions to pay for or offset the costs of the legislation.

In response to the CBC's letter, the White House convened a conference call with leaders of the Quad-Caucus, which included the Congressional Black Caucus, Congressional Hispanic Caucus, Congressional Asian Pacific American Caucus, and the Progressive Caucus. During the call with the president, these congressional leaders stressed the importance of expanding prevention and wellness services and the need for health equity provisions, such as data collection, workforce diversity, and community health workers. They emphasized that these provisions were necessary to address the root causes of the health inequities that disproportionately and detrimentally affected racial and ethnic minorities, women, rural Americans, and Americans in the US territories. According to Congresswoman Barbara Lee, the "discussion with President Obama was a useful and productive conversation."[5] The consensus was that the president appreciated their input and was taking their views seriously. The congressional Tri-Caucus iterated its commitment to working diligently on health reform to the president.

The National Working Group responded to the *New York Times* article by sending a letter to the White House urging the Obama administration to keep the data collection provisions in the health reform legislation. Fortunately, four days prior, the Institute of Medicine had released a report on August 31, 2009, titled *Race, Ethnicity, and Language Data: Standardization for Health Care Quality Improvement*, that bolstered arguments for more accurate and robust data collection and reporting. Later on, it all made sense why the White House was pressed to find provisions to cut that would reduce the costs of the bills.

One week after the White House had contacted the advocates on September 9, 2009, Obama spoke before a joint session of Congress and promised that his health reform proposal would not add to the deficit and would not cost more than $900 billion. This meant that the White House had to find ways to fulfill this promise, as did the congressional architects of the legislation who were also worried about public perception. Lawmakers were determined to meet the president's ceiling on the cost of the bill, while the working group was determined to continue arguing that their provisions would not only significantly reduce costs but also help to elevate the health of all Americans once implemented.

Having pushed back on attempts to undermine the health equity agenda that had been achieved in various reform bills, advocates faced another serious issue that needed to be immediately addressed. The US Commission on Civil Rights had submitted to President Obama and congressional leaders a letter criticizing inclusion of the workforce provisions in the House health reform bill (H.R. 3200) that prioritized giving grants to health professional schools to increase outreach to and training of underrepresented and disadvantaged groups. Health equity advocates were quite surprised because, as they had remembered, in 1999, the commission had released a report on health care disparities that underscored the importance of addressing this specific issue in public policy.[6] The Energy and Commerce staff asked the working group to meet with them immediately to discuss their reactions to the letter and what steps they should take to address this issue. Some staff thought that perhaps they should just negate these provisions, but that was not an option advocates would entertain. The working group pushed back and underscored the fact that, just ten years ago, this same commission had been pushing for just such a provision and now all of a sudden they were backpedaling. The working group argued that the provision was not advocating affirmative action policies but instead was urging schools to recognize that the increased diversity in patients warranted more culturally and linguistically appropriate care. How else could one deliver effective care without understanding the cultural and linguistic issues impacting it? Congressional staff then raised these arguments with the White House, and it was decided that they would be left in.

Making a Mark: The Bipartisan Health Reform Bill

In late September, the Senate Finance Committee continued debating its health reform proposal, the America's Healthy Future Act. During the fiery negotiations, the Senate Finance Committee convened a bipartisan group of senators, the "Gang of Six," which included three Republicans and three Democrats. The senators met thirty-one times to try to reach consensus. Senator Baucus, describing this process, stated, "We held exhaustive meetings. We met for more than 61 hours. We went the extra mile. And now, we've held an open and exhaustive markup. I put out the mark[up] and posted it on the Web on September 16. That was nearly a week before we started the markup. In a first for this Committee, we posted every amendment—all 564 of them—on the Web." The seven days of meetings leading up to the committee vote were long and stressful; no other bill under consideration by the Senate Finance Committee in the previous twenty-two years had demanded that amount of time for consideration.[7] At the end of the markup, the Senate Finance Committee approved the America's Healthy Future Act with a bipartisan 14-9 vote. The lone Republican voting in favor of the bill was Senator Olympia Snowe of Maine. In all, the committee had conducted seventy-nine roll call votes and adopted forty-one amendments. Meanwhile, on the House side, Speaker Nancy Pelosi promised that congressional members would have seventy-two hours—three days—to read their health reform bill before voting on it. Although some House members were upset by the time constraint, like Congresswoman Michele Bachmann (R-MN), who thought they should be given three months instead, most members did not argue that this was insufficient time to read a bill of that size.[8]

Advocates attempted to keep up with the lightning speed at which negotiations were taking place and to learn whether their priorities would be considered and included. The advocates saw this time as one of the last opportunities to have their public policy priorities included in the omnibus health reform legislation. They worked diligently to ensure that amendments that were proffered to advance health equity were adopted, including Senator Ben Cardin's amendment to transfer the Office of Minority Health at the Department of Health and Human Services from the Office of the Assistant Secretary to the Office of the Secretary, to establish six additional offices of minority health at various federal agencies, and to elevate the National Center on Minority Health and Health Disparities to an institute at the National Institutes of Health.

One stalwart health equity champion was state senator Shirley Nathan-Pulliam of Maryland. She demonstrated how lessons learned at the state level could help strengthen federal policies, and she worked with Cardin's office to develop this amendment. Through her work in the state legislature, she recognized an opportunity to elevate these entities at the federal level and, with Dr. Britt Weinstock, former director of the CBC Health Braintrust, and Priscilla Ross, former senior policy advisor to Cardin, pushed this amendment internally in Congress. Weinstock and Ross worked tirelessly into the early morning hours to educate and advocate for this amendment to ensure that it was considered and adopted. Even though Democrats led the House, the Senate, and the White House, surprisingly these two congressional staff had to fight to get their colleagues on the Democratic side to agree to include it in the health reform bill.

The working group also urged support for Senator Roland Burris's proposed amendment, the Health Entities Community Reinvestment Assistance Act, which would enable hospitals and other health care entities to appropriately respond to their local community health care needs and provide the technical assistance and training required to address critical disparities in health care. The amendment would strengthen the Senate Finance health reform bill's section on hospitals conducting community health needs assessments. It was significantly reduced to a couple sentences but was finally adopted by the committee along with Senator Cardin's amendments and ultimately included in the final bill.

During September, the National Working Group coordinated its largest event, a congressional briefing titled "Cost-Savings of Reducing Health Disparities in Health Reform." The lead-up to the event was stressful and time consuming, but because of a great deal of hard work and outstanding help and support, the working group put together an exceptional briefing. Their partners included the National Dental Association, WomenHeart: The National Coalition for Women with Heart Disease, the National Health Equity Coalition, Community Catalyst, National League for Nursing, National Korean-American Service and Education Consortium, and the Asian & Pacific Islander American Health Forum. Many different groups provided support either financially or by lending staff to develop signage, create fact sheets for distribution, or direct traffic flow. Members of the working group committed to sending out invitations to their contacts and following up with congressional offices. It was an excellent example of effective collaboration. The briefing would highlight the costs associated with health care inequalities among certain populations in the United States and include discussions of issues such as health workforce development, language access, health coverage, quality, and prevention.

One of the working group's biggest challenges was deciding which speakers to invite, but advocates agreed they should be as diverse as possible. They needed an expert on health disparities to give an overview, so they invited Dr. Norman Anderson, CEO of the American Psychological Association. They wanted to keep the White House closely linked to the event and hear how it was prioritizing health equity, so they invited Dr. Kavita Patel, director of policy in the White House Office of Public Engagement and Intergovernmental Affairs, who had championed health equity priorities at the White House. They also invited Dr. Carolyn Clancy, director of the Agency for Healthcare Research and Quality at Health and Human Services, whose agency had been instrumental in highlighting the disparities in the health system with their *National Healthcare Disparities Reports*.

The working group needed experts who understood the economic burden of health inequities to the United States, so they invited Drs. Brian Smedley, Len Nichols, and Timothy Waidmann to highlight these issues and unveil two seminal reports. The advocates also needed an expert from a group representing the civil rights organizations to highlight legal and policy issues impacting vulnerable groups, so they invited attorney David Goldberg, senior counsel of the Leadership Conference on Civil Rights. In addition to these policy experts, advocates wanted the briefing to include not only health policy experts with expertise on the national level but also experts on the state and local level, so they invited speakers such as Dr. Thomas Bornemann of the Carter Center and Marcos Pesquera of Adventist Healthcare's Center on Health Disparities, who were actually working within underresourced communities.

At the briefing, which was dedicated to the late Senator Kennedy, two landmark reports were unveiled on the costs of health disparities—one by the Urban Institute and one by the Joint Center for Political and Economic Studies.[9] The standing-room-only audience of more than 150 people included congressional staff from Democratic and Republican offices, representatives from the American Hospital Association, advocates from numerous health coalitions, and academic experts in health policy. The panelists addressed the issue of health equity from a national to a regional to a local level. During the event, it was challenging to keep presenters on message. Some of the talking points the working group wanted speakers to focus on were not adhered to, with some addressing their individual priorities instead of the broader ones of the National Working Group. But, despite those challenges, in the end the working group's message rang loud and clear, and the briefing was a great success.

Remembering the Forgotten Faces

A few days after the major congressional briefing, members of the working group attended the Congressional Black Caucus's fall 2009 Health Braintrust on September 25. The event was themed "Addressing the Forgotten Faces and Voices of Health Reform" and focused on health care reform, its impact on individuals, communities, providers, and businesses, and its role in health equity. Panelists included Nancy-Ann De-Parle, director of the White House Office of Health Reform. I was a panelist in the session "Opportunities in Health Care Reform: Filling in the Gaps around Scoring, Prevention and Health Equity" and delivered remarks about the role that health reform would play in reducing health disparities and improving the health of all communities affected by them. I laid out the case for addressing the less popular disparities issues, such as mental/behavioral and dental health. Previously, advocates focused on physical health disparities, and I was becoming frustrated that in the larger debate these lesser-addressed issues were being neglected.

At this conference, advocates told the story of a woman in her thirties with uncontrolled diabetes who lived with her two children and a relative in South Carolina. She did not qualify for Medicaid under South Carolina's guidelines because she had not yet been found disabled by the Social Security Administration. Since she had no treating physician, every time her blood sugar went too high or too low, she went to the local emergency department for treatment. She continually complained to the ED staff that she had a sore on her right foot that would not heal. No one evaluated her for this because they were concerned about getting her blood sugar under control. Every ED visit had notations of her unhealing sores but provided no treatment. Eventually, she insisted that the doctor look at the worsening sores on her foot. Once the doctor saw her foot, she was immediately admitted and the next day her leg was amputated below the knee. The surgeon could not remove all of the leg that needed to be removed and wanted to wait a few days because it would be too much of a shock to her system. The sores were so bad that, even with the amputation, osteomyelitis had set in, and before the next surgery could be performed, she died. Access to affordable health care would have enabled her to better manage her diabetes and could have saved her life.[10]

As health reform legislation continued moving forward, the working group forged ahead with their agenda to ensure that health equity was a major factor in the final bill. The working group drafted and sent another letter to Congress and the White House urging them to leave intact the health equity provisions secured in the health reform bills. These critical provisions addressed data collection, health care quality improvements, prevention and wellness, language access, and health workforce and infrastructure.

Within Reach

On October 29, 2009, Congressman John Dingell Jr. introduced the Affordable Health Care for America Act (H.R. 3962), the House's version of the health reform legislation. The bill was a revised version of an earlier, unsuccessful measure, the America's Affordable Health Choices Act (H.R. 3200), which had been introduced on July 14, 2009. The bill was revised to meet certain goals outlined in the president's September address to the joint session of Congress. Before House Democrats unveiled their health reform bill, they convened a meeting in the Capitol's basement for a final briefing with Speaker Pelosi and other leaders. All agreed at that time that the moment of compromise had finally arrived. No longer could the conservative and liberal factions of the caucus afford to continue fighting. The consensus at the meeting was that they had to pass the bill. The House of Representatives passed the Affordable Health Care for America Act on November 7, 2009, in a 220-215 vote.[11] One Republican, Congressman Joseph Cao of Louisiana, voted in favor of the bill. If the Senate would go on to pass its own bill, the House and Senate bills would have to be reconciled into one document and voted on again.

During this suspenseful time, health equity proponents took notice of a groundbreaking report that was released on November 5, 2009, *Ready, Willing, and Unable to Serve*, by Mission: Readiness, a nonprofit organization led by prominent senior retired military leaders, including two former chairmen of the Joint Chiefs of Staff in conjunction with the US Department of Defense. According to the report, "approximately 75 percent of young people aged seventeen to twenty-four are unable to enlist in the military because they fail to graduate from high school, have a criminal record, or are physically unfit." The report noted that one in ten young people could not join because they had at least one prior conviction for a felony or serious misdemeanor. It also found that approximately 30 percent of young people were rejected because they were too overweight to join the military, and other individuals were unqualified because of visual or hearing impairments or mental health issues. To bolster their arguments in support of health reform, and more specifically, prioritizing health equity, advocates used this report to highlight the national security implications of poor health and inequities in health status given the changing demographics. Just as health equity champions had done in 1946 when they raised the national security implications of increasing mental health conditions impacting young people, health equity champions adopted that playbook to show how much more dire things were in the country now.

In 1946, policy makers were concerned that 20 percent of young people were unfit to serve in the military. In 2009, 75 percent of young people were unfit to serve in the military, a drastic and alarming increase. With birth rates of racial and ethnic minorities expected to outnumber white birth rates in the next few years, policy makers could no longer punt the issue of elevating health equity into the future, advocates argued. In the next two decades, many of these minority population groups who had long struggled with poorer health and inequities would be old enough to serve and, therefore, would be unable to owing to their health status.

In the Senate, Majority Leader Harry Reid and Senators Max Baucus, Tom Harkin, and Chris Dodd worked together to merge the Finance Committee's health reform bill, the America's Healthy Future Act, with the bill passed by the Health Education Labor and Pensions Committee, the Affordable Health Choices Act. Since the Constitution requires all revenue-related bills to originate in the House, the Senate adopted H.R. 3590, a bill regarding housing tax breaks for service members, because it was first passed by the House as a revenue-related modification to the Internal Revenue Code.[12] The Senate then revised the content of the bill, using it as their vehicle for health reform legislation. The result was the Patient Protection and Affordable Care Act, which on November 19, 2009, was sent to the Senate floor for debate. Republicans were eager to drag out this debate for weeks, if not longer, while Democrats were eager to have the health reform bill passed and enacted into law by the end of the following month.

Republicans used their time to question whether the bill would actually reduce health care costs to Americans. They questioned the legitimacy of the cost of the health reform bill itself, which the nonpartisan Congressional Budget Office now concluded would equate to approximately $850 billion. Republicans also questioned the methodology for arriving at that figure, as well as policy decisions or tactics used by Democrats to ensure the bill would not exceed $1 trillion in costs. Democrats, by contrast, discussed key provisions that were included in the bill and argued for additional policies they strongly believed should be included. They also argued for the continued inclusion of a public health insurance option that Americans could choose when purchasing health insurance coverage in the proposed health insurance exchange or marketplace. Democrats argued that reforming health care would improve the economy and emphasized that the health reform bill included provisions that would reduce the deficit and reduce costs to both state and federal governments while increasing access to health care and improving health outcomes.

On December 24, 2009—Christmas Eve morning—the Senate convened a vote for the Patient Protection and Affordable Care Act. The vote was the culmination of twenty-five consecutive days of intense debate, the second-longest run in Senate history, and the first Christmas Eve Senate session since 1985. Before the vote, Senate Majority Leader Reid asserted, "Opponents of this bill have used every trick in the book to delay this day. And yet, here we are, minutes away from doing what many have tried, but none has ever achieved. We are here because facts will always defeat fear. And though one might slow the speed of progress, its force cannot be stopped."[13]

With Senator Kirk seated, Democrats once again had the sixty votes needed to pass their health reform bill, but there was no guarantee that all the Democratic senators would vote in its favor. Just as they did years earlier with the Clinton health reform proposal, the National Federation of Independent Business and other probusiness lobbying groups worked determinedly to prevent the Obama health reform proposal from gaining any further momentum. Certain senators had leveraged their votes to gain concessions for their states and key stakeholders. Senator Joseph Lieberman of Connecticut, a former Democrat turned Independent, refused to vote in favor of any bill that included a public option that would compete with the private insurers in his state. Senator Ben Nelson (D-NE) agreed to vote in favor of the law only if Nebraska's Medicaid expansion was fully paid for by the federal government and the law included language restricting federal funding from paying for abortion coverage. Senator Bill Nelson (D-FL) demanded protections for Medicare Advantage plans in Florida, and Senator Mary Landrieu (D-LA) was promised $300 million for Louisiana's Medicaid program, which came to be referred to as the "Louisiana Purchase."[14]

In the end, Reid was able to cut enough deals to gain the support of every member of the Democratic caucus. On Christmas Eve morning, the Patient Protection and Affordable Care Act passed on a 60-39 party-line vote. Shortly after the vote, President Obama declared, "We are now finally poised to deliver on the promise of real, meaningful health insurance reform that will bring additional security and stability to the American people." As tough as it was to pass this bill with the fierce winds of opposition continually blowing, Senate Minority Leader Mitch McConnell vowed after the vote to continue fighting against health reform: "The public is on our side. This fight is not over."[15]

After the December vote on health reform in the Senate, Scott Brown won Senator Kennedy's Senate seat in the Massachusetts special election. When Brown, a Tea Party-backed Republican who ran on a platform of opposing health reform, won the election, many feared the opportunity to pass comprehensive health reform had been lost to history. The January 19, 2010, special election was between Brown and Martha Coakley, the state's attorney general, who had been widely expected to win. Instead, Brown won, with 52 percent of the vote. The election result stunned the nation, especially proponents of health reform. Massachusetts had always voted reliably Democratic, so this was supposed to have been a relatively safe seat. The political ramifications of such a liberal-leaning state electing a candidate who strongly opposed health reform were major, in particular because Massachusetts had earlier enacted its own health insurance reforms. Again, health equity proponents were faced with how the political determinants of health, particularly voting, could jeopardize the progress made in advancing their agenda.

Brown's victory left Democrats just short of the sixty votes needed for a filibuster-proof majority in the Senate, which meant that Republicans would now be able to obstruct the progress and passage of any bill. Soon after the election results, Senator Jim Webb of Virginia, a moderate Democrat, called on his Senate colleagues to hold off on voting on the health reform legislation until Senator-elect Brown was sworn into office. He firmly believed that the election was a referendum on health reform. Reid decided to hold off on the vote until Brown was sworn in, stating, "We're going to wait until the new senator arrives until we do anything more on health care."[16]

The strategy all along had been to pass two health reform bills—one in the Senate and one in the House—that could be merged together in conference. The combined bill would then be voted on again; however, with Brown's victory, it was now unlikely that a health reform bill could make it through the Senate. Democrats therefore decided to avoid a second Senate vote by having the House pass the bill that the Senate had passed on Christmas Eve a month prior. However, some House Democrats had concerns about passing the Senate bill. Although both bills contained many similar priorities, some major provisions differentiated the two. The House bill, for example, had a public option and imposed taxes on wealthy individuals, while the Senate bill did not have a public option and taxed only expensive health insurance plans. House members were also wary of passing the Senate bill, especially during an election year, because of the inclusion of certain provisions that were deemed kickbacks for various states, including Florida, Louisiana, and Nebraska. Whether House members' expressed discontent with the Senate-passed bill was a political strategy to gain some concessions and include priorities from their own bill, it was clear that these lawmakers would not accept the Senate-passed plan without some changes.

Speaker Pelosi, understanding the incredible and rare opportunity before the House, seized the moment and went about implementing a strategy that would prove successful in regaining her caucus's faith and their acceptance of the Senate version of the health care bill. She decided to use a reconciliation bill, which would require only a majority vote by both chambers, to address her colleagues' concerns with the Senate-approved bill. The result of Pelosi's work was the Health Care and Education Reconciliation Act, which would make several changes to the Patient Protection and Affordable Care Act. It would get rid of many of the concessions given to certain states, such as Nebraska's Medicaid expansion kickback. It would also increase tax credits for purchasing insurance, reduce the penalty for not purchasing insurance, provide full reimbursement for doctors who care for Medicaid patients, and many other amendments. Although opponents of the law tried in vain to argue to the parliamentarian why certain provisions of the ACA were not germane to the reconciliation procedure, with the strategy executed and House Democrats on board, the stage was now set for the House to vote on the Patient Protection and Affordable Care Act. As negotiations proceeded the enactment of health reform legislation was not just within sight but within reach.

There was a great deal of tension and concern among health equity advocates regarding the meaning of Brown's election for health reform and their work to advance health equity. One year after the presidential election, they were finally seeing the light at the end of the tunnel, and now all that progress was in jeopardy. They got calls and emails from advocates concerned about the health equity provisions in the House and Senate health reform legislation. They responded that advocates could not remain quiet about their support for the health disparities provisions that had taken a lot of effort to secure and that it was crucial not to give up at this point. The momentum that they had seen from congressional health reformers seemed to be slowing now. This alarmed health equity leaders who were frustrated by the hesitation or second guessing of congressional champions on whether to continue pushing health reform.

They urged advocates to contact their members of Congress, especially leadership in the House and Senate, voicing their strong support for moving the Senate-passed bill, which included provisions aimed at reducing health disparities and improving the health status of all population groups. They contacted lawmakers, urging them to pass health reform quickly before the window of opportunity closed, and reminded these leaders that their provisions would potentially save more than $60 billion a year in direct health care expenditures and countless lives. While their advocacy campaign continued in high gear, Families USA, the Raising Women's Voices coalition, Community Catalyst, and the National Partnership for Women and Families, which were members of the working group, including approximately fifty academics from across the country, sent out action alerts or circulated their own letters to Congress urging them to not delay passing health reform. Instead, advocates argued, Congress should focus their energies on moving health reform forward to its needed enactment and stressed the belief that now was the time to speak up before it was too late.

Health reformers in Congress and the White House had been proposing several strategies to move forward with health reform. One major strategy debated by the White House and congressional champions involved moving away from comprehensive health care reform legislation to piecemeal legislation. Another major strategy that was increasingly gaining support involved using the "more popular and less controversial" components of the two health care reform bills. This ambiguous strategy was concerning to health equity advocates because they were not sure whether health equity provisions would fall into that category and thus be included in the final bill.

In the weeks leading up to the final vote on the combined health reform proposal, they continued to urge congressional champions of health reform and health equity to stay the course and keep the package intact. They then started seeing senior officials in the administration and Congress becoming more vocal and agreeing that approach was the best alternative in light of the circumstances. More Democratic lawmakers soon argued that they believed it was crucial to pass a bill and show some success after negotiating for more than a year. And in March 2010, on the weekend prior to the vote on the Patient Protection and Affordable Care Act, the National Working Group organized massive final grassroots efforts to urge lawmakers to vote in support of health reform.

Finalizing and Passing the Policy: Maneuvering the Final Aspect of the Political Determinants of Health

The American Medical Association announced on the Friday before the final vote that it endorsed the revised health reform legislation.

According to the president of the AMA, "This is certainly not the bill we would have written, but we cannot let the perfect be the enemy of the good."[17] The AMA had earlier announced support for the House version of the bill that passed in November and the Senate version that passed in December.

Despite the Democrats' control of the House, the votes to pass the bill were never guaranteed. The intense congressional negotiations over health reform had led to increased partisanship and gridlock, limiting Congress's ability to introduce and pass other major bills. House members were particularly worried about casting a "dangerous" vote and of potential backlash from their constituents. The White House expended considerable time and energy hosting meetings with wavering Democrats in the House and all but begged them to vote in favor of the Patient Protection and Affordable Care Act. Leading unions were not happy with the final package but decided to lend their support to the administration and congressional lawmakers. Pro-life advocates urged conservative anti-abortion Democrats to vote against the package. The White House was eager to allay any concerns these Blue Dog Democrats may have had, and Obama promised them that no abortions would be funded under the act.

On Sunday, March 21, 2010, arguably the most emotionally riveting and the pivotal day in the health reform debate, the House of Representatives was scheduled to vote at 1 p.m. on the health reform package that had previously been voted on by the Senate a few months earlier on Christmas Eve. The actual vote would not take place until much later that evening. On that day, the pressure from opponents of health reform intensified, with protesters active outside the Capitol. While congressional proponents were walking to the Capitol to cast their historic votes, many were taunted, vilified, and even spat on. Congressman John Lewis (D-GA), a strong proponent of health reform even during the Clinton negotiations, when recalling his most memorable time during the health reform negotiations, stated that it was the march to the Capitol to cast his historic vote that he remembers most fondly.[18] It is a day neither he nor other congressional champions will soon forget. Among the ranks of advocates were many supporters of the health reform bill urging the lawmakers not to stand down but to be courageous and vote in support of this bill even though it might not be popular. No matter what either side was advocating for, the final votes were sure to be extremely close.

That Sunday at 2 p.m., the House of Representatives convened to vote on the health reform bill. The vote carried with it major political ramifications for the future. All day long, the Representatives argued over H.R. 3590 and H.R. 4872, the health reform package. Lewis, a civil rights icon who had helped spearhead the historic civil rights march from Selma to Montgomery, urged his colleagues not to be fearful and to "answer the call of history." In a passionate and stern manner, House Minority Leader John Boehner (R-OH) warned his colleagues that voting in favor of the act would be "denying the will of the American people."[19]

A little after 10:45 that night the announcement came that the bill had finally passed the House by the incredibly slim margin of 219-212—just seven votes—with no Republicans voting in favor of the bill. All 178 Republicans opposed it, along with 34 Democrats.[20] The vote had been agonizingly close, right up to the last minute, but the results were now clear. Health reform champions inside and outside of Congress that night erupted in cheers. Opponents of health reform were more subdued and promised to use every resource and tactic they could to ensure that the bill would never be implemented.

On March 23, 2010, President Obama signed into law the Patient Protection and Affordable Care Act:

> After a century of striving, after a year of debate, after a historic vote, health care reform is no longer an unmet promise. It is the law of the land. It is the law of the land.
>
> And although it may be my signature that's affixed to the bottom of this bill, it was your work, your commitment, your unyielding hope that made this victory possible. When the special interests deployed an army of lobbyists, an onslaught of negative ads, to preserve the status quo, you didn't give up. You hit the phones and you took to the streets. You mobilized and you organized. You turned up the pressure and you kept up the fight.[21]

It was a groundbreaking piece of legislation, which advocates hoped would bring coverage to more than thirty-two million uninsured Americans. It materialized because advocates were "unwilling to postpone" the creation, passage, and implementation of the country's first inclusive and equitable health law. The law contained many provisions concerning health equity and the elimination of health disparities, and it was the most significant and inclusive federal effort directly addressing health disparities in the country's history.[22] However, though the Affordable Care Act had finally been enacted and all this promise had been achieved, its proponents had to temper their celebrations. They would soon be forced to tackle many obstacles in the path of the ACA's implementation.

As advocates and lawmakers would soon realize, getting the law enacted was the shockingly easy part. The hardest part was yet to come as health equity proponents would soon learn how the political determinants of health operate simultaneously in ways that mutually reinforce one another to shape opportunities that either advance health equity or exacerbate health inequities. This is not a linear process, but one that is influenced and responsive to the events of the day.

6

Growing Pains
Tackling the Political Determinants of Health Inequities during a Challenging Period

> We choose to go to the moon in this decade and do the other things, not because they are easy, but because they are hard, because that goal will serve to organize and measure the best of our energies and skills, because that challenge is one that we are willing to accept, one we are unwilling to postpone, and one which we intend to win.—*President John F. Kennedy, Rice University*

From 2008 to 2016, voters allowed a fundamental shift in health policy with the election of President Obama, almost 150 years after the first major health equity legislation was passed, signed into law, and dismantled just seven years afterward. A majority of voters in 2008 put in place a government that would develop a comprehensive health equity-focused policy—the Affordable Care Act—fix the economic and financial engines of the country, and tackle disparities in our educational system, among other significant reforms. Once the new government convened, advocates who championed health equity took lessons from history and successfully traversed the political minefield that had long deterred prior health equity attempts.

The Power of Political Determinants of Health Post-Obama Administration: Voting, Government, Policy

Eight years after voters allowed a fundamental shift to occur in health policy, there was a different set of political determinants in play, with an unusually highly contentious election, a new government opposed to addressing racial and ethnic disparities, LGBTQ+ disparities, immigrant health issues, and climate change. There were also attempts to undermine health equity-focused policies that had been established by Republican and Democratic administrations since President Ronald Reagan. The

2016 elections marked a watershed moment for health equity, with the election of Donald J. Trump, who had vowed to shred ObamaCare to pieces and reverse other Obama administration health equity-focused policies.

Before the 2016 election, the Affordable Care Act had survived four national elections and many brushes with death, proving that it had more lives than a cat. It is true that there had been seventeen successful legislative efforts that repealed or modified certain provisions of the ACA before the election took place, but those efforts were relatively minor, failing to strike at the heart and guts of the law. However, an unexpected upset occurred in the 2016 elections when Hillary Clinton, the Democratic nominee who was long-expected to win, lost to a man who few people believed stood a real chance of beating the more seasoned politician among the two. Until this time, there was always a Democrat in the White House to prevent the Republican-led Congress from overturning the law, but now with Republicans controlling the executive and legislative branches of government, ObamaCare proponents were concerned about the act's future.

There was always a chance that the political winds could shift and support for the law could diminish as a result. For now, proponents of the ACA would have to wait and see whether the president and congressional Republicans would finally succeed in eliminating the health reform law and repeating one of the nation's most unfortunate events: when it succeeded in passing the most comprehensive federal law intended to address the social determinants of health but saw its demise after seven years as health equity advocates lost the fight to continue beating back attempts to repeal it. After the 2016 presidential elections, ACA proponents regrouped to determine the best course of action to protect the health law, given the political circumstances, engaging in the four-step process of due diligence to ascertain the challenges and opportunities before them; to negotiate with stakeholders and advocates of the law to develop consensus around the best strategy; to understand the internal and external strengths that would come to bear in moving forward, including the commercial interests, the government investment value, and the political interests; and to try to preserve as much of the law as possible given the political quagmire they faced.

Voting as a Political Determinant of Health

On Tuesday, November 8, 2016, the world waited with great anticipation to see who would become the forty-fifth president of the United

States. The choices were Hillary Clinton, the lawyer, former First Lady, and career politician, and Donald Trump, the billionaire real-estate mogul with no political experience. Democrats had expected huge wins: the election of Clinton as the first female president of the United States and the return of the US Senate to Democratic control. If lucky, and with an expected Democratic sweep, it was possible they could even regain a majority in the House of Representatives.

The election cycle had been long, fiery, and highly charged, and polls in the days leading up to November 8 had assured most people that Hillary Clinton would win. As early results started coming in from polling places on the East Coast, Hillary Clinton appeared to be the front-runner. But things quickly changed. Clinton was losing critical electoral votes in the Midwest, which had long been a reliably Democratic stronghold, along with swing states, such as Florida and North Carolina. Data would later show a significant decline in African American and Hispanic turnout, two groups that stood to lose if the Obama era health law was successfully repealed or undermined. Shortly after midnight, Trump was declared the president-elect, pulling off one of the greatest upsets in US political history and capturing the highest office in the world. People on both sides of the political aisle were caught off guard, stunned, or in awe of the result. Republicans scrambled to assess and leverage the opportunities this presented, while Democrats scrambled to assess and effectually respond to the challenges that were ahead.

Government as a Political Determinant of Health

From a health equity perspective, the implications of this election were clear: advocates would now be consumed with fighting to preserve the gains they had made in public policy and law. They would be playing more defensive advocacy. The crowning policy achievement for health equity leaders—the Affordable Care Act—would now experience its closest brush with death, and other critical health equity-focused policies would be in jeopardy if campaign promises were actually kept. Undoubtedly, the 2016 election marked a critical juncture for health equity in the United States. Would the new government fully commit to implementing existing health, education, housing, transportation, food, economic, climate, and civil rights policies, while advancing new policies intended to create and sustain a more equitable society? Or would it reverse course by initiating new policies which lead to increasing health disparities?

During the transition period, before Trump's inauguration, proponents of the Affordable Care Act pondered what they could have done differently to change Trump's position on completely getting rid of Obama-Care. Many wondered why had this election gone off the rails. Did the Obama administration not do enough to tout the benefits and accomplishments of the Affordable Care Act? Had proponents of the law not done enough to get the word out on the serious impact of repeal? Or had advocates become too complacent because the bill had survived dozens of legislative challenges?

How was it that the ACA—a health law that had benefited all geographic, socioeconomic, racial, gender, and age groups—was now precariously hanging in the balance? During the campaign, it was hard for many health equity leaders to wrap their heads around how so many people who had benefited from the health reform law could allow their blind contempt for President Obama to make them vote against their own health and well-being. More than twenty million people had gotten health insurance coverage under the ACA—two-thirds of whom had a high school education or less and had voted overwhelmingly for a candidate who had explicitly declared his opposition to the health law and vowed to shred it to pieces.

Many ACA proponents quickly concluded that these questions would likely never be fully answered to their satisfaction and would not change the reality that they were under new management. After the election, their focus would now be spent on changing the new president's mind about repealing the Affordable Care Act, as well as Republican members of Congress. "Repeal and replace" had turned from a campaign slogan into a legislative directive, one that, over the coming months, would switch from "repeal only" to "repeal and delay" before coming back full circle. In determining how to best leverage the political determinants of health once the new government convened, to save not only the Affordable Care Act but also other health equity-focused policies, advocates decided—once it was clear that Trump was set on repealing the law—to focus their efforts on building grassroots momentum and to work on persuading legislators that voters did not want the law repealed.

Policy as a Political Determinant of Health

During the 115th Congress as efforts to repeal the ACA came to a climax, advocates wrestled with the ill-informed and exaggerated talking points of politicians who argued that they wanted to repeal and replace the ACA with a better policy. After several replacement proposals were introduced, a majority of experts, both liberal and conservative, as well as the nonpartisan Congressional Budget Office, which analyzes bills to determine their economic impact, found that the Republican bills would have increased costs and the number of uninsured people in the United States. It was clear that the calls for repeal were solely meant to dismantle Obama's greatest accomplishment or score political wins. According to the *Washingtonian*,[1] former House Majority Leader Eric Cantor (R-VA) said he never believed Republicans could repeal ObamaCare under President Obama despite using repeal as a rallying cry in the 2014 midterm elections. "To give the impression that if Republicans were in control of the House and Senate, that we could do that when Obama was still in office. . . . I never believed it." The article continues that it was a stunning admission from a former member of the party leadership—that the linchpin of GOP electoral strategy for the better part of a decade was a fantasy, a flame continually fanned solely because, when it came to midterm elections, it worked. But with Republicans now controlling the executive and legislative branches of government, the question remained, Would they, after years of vilifying ObamaCare, muster the will and garner the votes to finally accomplish their number one health policy priority?

Trump was inaugurated president on January 20, 2017, and his first act was to sign an executive order that "minimizes the economic burden" of ObamaCare. This was the moment when health equity advocates' worst fears seemed to be coming true. In its seventh year, the most *comprehensive and inclusive health legislation* ever passed by Congress was seemingly doomed to meet a fate similar to that of its precursor, the Freedmen's Bureau Act 150 years before.

Trump's executive order required the secretary of Health and Human Services and other agencies to waive, defer, grant exemptions from, or delay any requirement of ObamaCare that would impose a fiscal burden. This order came a week after the House of Representatives passed a bill that was the first step in a two-step process of repealing the law. Less than one year before that, the Affordable Care Act was nearly dismantled when congressional Republicans used a fast-track legislative tool known as reconciliation to pass H.R. 3762, Restoring Americans' Healthcare Freedom Reconciliation Act of 2015, which was sent to President Obama's desk with only a simple majority in the Senate. Obama, of course, vetoed the bill on January 8, 2016.

While the ACA had come back from the grave this time, with a new captain at the helm, future efforts to repeal the health law were expected to be less challenging. From the first day of the new administration, Republicans set out to roll back benefits of the ACA gained by millions of Americans. Fast-forward a few months into Trump's presidency and the entire country had been on a bumpy ride on the repeal-and-replace express. Some of the policy ideas Republicans proposed included Medicaid block grants; phasing out ACA Medicaid expansion over several years, timed to end after the 2020 presidential election; increasing contribution limits on Health Savings Accounts, which are mostly used by higher earners; selling insurance across state lines; eliminating the Prevention and Public Health Fund; striking the Section 1557 nondiscrimination provision; "repeal now, replace later"; and rolling out the replacement in phases. Regardless of the angle, the Congressional Budget Office showed that all of the major Republican proposals would kick as few as fifteen million and as many as thirty-two million people off insurance rolls over the coming decade.[2]

While it has been no surprise that Republicans have thrown their full force behind repealing and replacing ObamaCare, the increase in public interest and support for the law was a game changer. As English philosopher Francis Bacon once argued, "In order for the light to shine so brightly, the darkness must be present." Perhaps the 2016 election and the subsequent challenges were a blessing in disguise for the landmark health care law, for when the statute was in serious jeopardy, people started watching more carefully and making efforts to understand what was really at stake with a repeal of the ACA. Prior to 2017, it had been relatively difficult for advocates to inform the public about the merits of the health law. Opponents had outspent proponents of this policy, fifteen to one in advertising and other initiatives to put the law in a negative light. However, immediately following the election of Trump, reports emerged that ObamaCare enrollments had surged despite the law's uncertainty. In December 2016, enrollments were up nearly half a million from the year before, mostly from states that Trump carried in the election, such as Texas, North Carolina, Florida, Georgia, and Pennsylvania.[3]

The Power and Challenges of Advocacy

Weeks after Trump was inaugurated, polls showed that a majority of registered voters supported keeping and improving the ACA rather than repealing and replacing the law. Interestingly, most polls since the election showed that ObamaCare was more popular than Trump, Republicans, and Democrats.[4] This renewed engagement came to life after advocates were determined not to allow history to repeat itself with the repeal of a major health policy that had taken generations to realize. They adopted strategies from opponents of the ACA, including attending town hall meetings packed to the rafters, organizing several demonstrations, and engaging in impromptu protests in and around Capitol Hill throughout every effort to repeal the law.

The public disapproval and protests demonstrated to health equity advocates that there was hope in saving the ACA because what was actually happening in people's lives—in doctors' offices, nursing homes, hospitals, and rehabilitative treatment facilities—took precedence over talking points made popular on the campaign trail. Oddly, it also showed that many Americans literally did not understand that ObamaCare and the ACA were the same, and they raised their voices when they realized their health care might be taken away.

The president's and Republicans' failure to repeal the ACA lies mostly in the unprecedented speed, exclusivity, and level of secrecy involved in the process, where very few health care stakeholders had been given an ownership interest in the legislation. To his credit, Trump took a page from Obama's playbook by getting started on health reform immediately and allowing legislators to take the lead on drafting legislation. However, to his detriment, failing to understand the government investment value in passing the ACA in the first place or the commercial interests that were at stake and enshrouding the process in secrecy was a faulty tactic from the Clinton era. The lesson to be learned in both scenarios is simple: success is found in an inclusive, thoughtful, and public process. Ignoring this lesson, especially when developing health policies, results in the stark revelation, as Trump admitted afterward, "nobody knew healthcare could be so complicated."

In an address to the US Senate on July 25, 2017, Republican senator John McCain, who was battling glioblastoma and had voted against repealing the Affordable Care Act, reminded his colleagues about the importance of compromise and civility, arguing,

> Our healthcare insurance system is a mess. We all know it, those who support Obamacare and those who oppose it. Something has to be done. We Republicans have looked for a way to end it and replace it with something else without paying a terrible political price. We haven't found it yet, and I'm not sure we will. . . . What have we to lose by trying to work together to find those solutions? We're not getting much done apart. I don't think any of us

feels very proud of our incapacity. Merely preventing your political opponents from doing what they want isn't the most inspiring work. There's greater satisfaction in respecting our differences but not letting them prevent agreements that don't require abandonment of core principles, agreements made in good faith that help improve lives and protect the American people.

Throughout the entire repeal process, Trump stayed out of the weeds, used very general superlatives to describe forthcoming legislation, and then turned around to describe bills he had previously supported as "mean" once public opposition to those bills intensified. Moreover, when the efforts seemed to be at a standstill, he took to Twitter to single out members of his own party, called meetings at the White House to urge senators to vote "yes," and publicly suggested alternatives that had not been vetted with Republican leadership. Overall, it was a poorly coordinated repeal effort by the White House, which may have possibly also helped ObamaCare proponents protect the act.

Not long after the Senate's failure to pass a repeal bill, Senate Majority Leader Mitch McConnell and Trump started pointing fingers. Approximately two weeks after the GOP's failure to repeal the health law, McConnell blamed the failure on Trump's political inexperience, which led him to set unreasonable timelines: "Our new president, of course, has not been in this line of work before. And I think he had excessive expectations about how quickly things happen in the democratic process."[5] McConnell further stated, "So part of the reason I think people feel we're underperforming is because too many artificial deadlines—unrelated to the reality of the complexity of legislating—may not have been fully understood." Trump, along with several loyalists, quickly lashed out via Twitter, arguing that Republicans had had seven years to repeal the Affordable Care Act and insinuated that this was more than enough time to get it done.

The Consequences of the Political Determinants of Health Post-Obama Administration

While the repeal-and-replace legislative strategy largely failed to repeal the ACA in its entirety, the Trump administration and the Republican-controlled Congress eliminated the individual mandate in their tax-reform legislation. The Trump administration was also diligently engaged in efforts to further undermine the law administratively by minimizing enrollment in health plans sold in the health insurance marketplace and creating regulatory instability by refusing to fund cost-

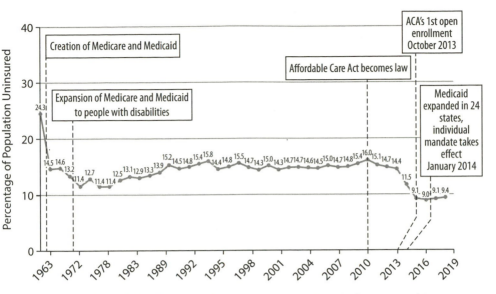

US uninsured rate during Obama and Trump administrations. Council of Economic Advisors, 2014, and National Center for Health Statistics, "National Health Interview Survey," January–September 2015.

sharing subsidies. ObamaCare enrollment in 2016 was on track to surpass previous years but dropped off following the transition in White House administrations. The Trump administration pulled ads that were promoting ACA enrollment, arguing that the decision was designed to cut costs, but it was later discovered that the administration was using those funds to run negative ads against the ACA. The administration targeted additional funding that was also intended to promote ACA enrollment, clawing back 90 percent of the funding for the navigators who were charged with providing information about the health insurance marketplace and helping consumers sign up for health insurance coverage. The negative impact of these administrative efforts have, for the first time since the ACA's health insurance marketplace began enrolling consumers in October 2013, led to lower enrollments. After reaching its lowest uninsured rate at the end of 2016, two years into the Trump administration, the uninsured rate in the United States increased significantly according to estimates provided by the US Census Bureau, Gallup, and the Urban Institute.

The level of opposition to bolstering minority health, eliminating health disparities, and advancing health equity under the Trump administration is higher than we have seen in the United States in generations.

Opponents, either because of their ignorance, disdain, or apathy, managed to roll back gains made in public policy to advance health equity, essentially preventing disenfranchised groups of people an opportunity to achieve their optimal level of health and become productive citizens. While this chapter has focused on the backlash against the ACA, there were additional battles to prevent the termination of key health equity policies, programs, and initiatives, including a major disagreement over the HHS Strategic Plan FY 2018-2022, which negated references to health equity, racial and ethnic disparities, disability disparities, and LGBTQ+ disparities. The previous plan, which was developed and implemented under the Obama administration, had specifically prioritized these issues.

The Trump administration attempted to prevent the federal government from collecting and reporting race and ethnicity data, recouping funding intended for navigators, expanding cheap short-term plans, and shortening the enrollment period that resulted in estimated millions of Americans losing health insurance coverage. In addition, health equity leaders had to push back against Trump administration efforts to close and reorganize the Office of Minority Health at the Department of Health and Human Services, as well as some of the other agency offices of minority health, which were established or codified into law by the Affordable Care Act. Other attempts were made to erode Section 1557, the antidiscrimination provision of the Affordable Care Act, and led to a sweeping new proposed rule in the third year of the Trump administration to substantially repeal most of the Obama administration's original rule, which expanded protections for LGBTQ+ individuals, people with limited English proficiency, and other vulnerable populations. Health equity proponents also had to contend with proposals to reorganize the National Institutes of Health's institutes and centers to focus on highest priority research, categorizing health disparities research as lower priority. The US Census Bureau's consideration of a citizenship question brought back memories of when the federal government used census data to round up innocent Japanese Americans and put them in internment camps. Health equity leaders were concerned about the implications of this political determinant (a citizenship question) as a tool to further disenfranchise certain groups. Advocates were also concerned about the health ramifications of Trump's withdrawal from the Paris Climate agreement and his refusal to acknowledge the effects of climate change.

Why Advocacy Matters No Matter What the Period

While mostly unsuccessful, these attempts would have further exacerbated the inequities in our country if advocates had not mobilized to thwart these political actions by collectively drafting and sending letters to the administration, initiating public comment writing campaigns opposing changes that would undermine health equity, meeting with administration officials to discuss the implications of the proposed policies, leveraging the power of the media to raise awareness of issues, and working with a bipartisan group of congressional members to put the brakes on policy changes that would have hurt health equity efforts. The Trump administration repeatedly sought the demise of America's most inclusive and equitable health law. Vice President Mike Pence even stated that the president would keep fighting until a bill to repeal and replace ObamaCare is sent to his desk. Although that may not happen in Trump's first term owing to the 2018 midterm elections, which elevated Democrats to the majority in the House of Representatives, repealing and replacing the ACA could happen through other avenues.

Unlike the Freedmen's Bureau Act, which Congress ultimately terminated, there are multiple levels and levers from which to eliminate or prevent a policy agenda from thriving. Consider, for example, the post-Civil War civil rights cases that were continuously brought before the judicial branch, urging the courts to strike down legislative advancements of civil rights. They were ultimately struck down. It would take another hundred years before civil rights advocates in the next century managed to pass legislation mirrored after those original policies. As is the case with multiple state attorneys general who have initiated one lawsuit after another seeking the demise of the ACA, the opposition to policies advancing health equity has been unrelenting.

The rollback of key health equity initiatives, as well as attempted efforts to undermine programs and policies focused on addressing health inequities, should alarm all health equity proponents. The rollback of health equity initiatives repeats similar efforts that past generations of Americans have witnessed and has led to erasing some of the gains that have been made in prioritizing health equity. Consequently, if history is any indication, it will take a groundswell of public pressure to change the nation's partial commitment to health equality to a full commitment to health equality. Unlike in the past, when health care was not the top issue on voters' minds, today health care is the centerpiece of voters' concerns.

More voters want increased scrutiny of health care and pharmaceutical drug pricing, reform of health care payments, and universal health care, single-payer, or "Medicare for All" to bolster access to quality care and treatments.

In June 2019, a significant number of members of the American Medical Association came very close to overturning the association's long-standing opposition to single-payer health care. Members pushed for the AMA's House of Delegates to support Medicare for All, which resulted in 53 percent against the idea but a remarkable 47 percent in support, demonstrating single-payer advocates' impact on bolstering this health policy agenda. During this challenging period for health equity, there were some bright spots: election of the first African American female president of the AMA, Dr. Patrice Harris, who was deeply committed to advancing health equity, as well as other health equity leaders at other associations; bipartisan congressional support for existing health equity-focused policies; and attention to bolstering behavioral health and expanding delivery and payment system reforms by the Trump administration. However, these gains are overshadowed by the onslaught of attacks against existing laws that were primarily focused on achieving health equity for all.

Coupled with the seemingly unending fight to increase access and improve health care quality, another equally important fight to address critical areas of policy impacting our ability to live longer and fruitful lives were the social, environmental, economic, and behavioral health determinants. These, too, required focused advocacies and the application of an equity lens to policies that affect those areas, which, in turn, impact health equity. Unless society begins to employ a new ecological and multidisciplinary approach and understand and leverage the political determinants of health, health inequities may get worse before they get better.

7

The Future of Health Equity Begins and Ends with the Political Determinants of Health

The price one pays for pursuing any profession, or calling, is an intimate knowledge of its ugly side.—*James Baldwin,* Nobody Knows My Name: More Notes of a Native Son

Health equity is the great unfinished business of our society. It has eluded the United States and other countries, owing in large part to vexing political determinants undergirded by structural racism, misogyny, and other forms of inequality. As Dr. Gary D. Nelson, president of the Healthcare Georgia Foundation and a notable expert on population health, often reminds leaders, health equity, broadly defined, is both a process and an outcome. It is both a journey and a destination. The voyage is disruptive, uncomfortable, and threatens a system that despises major reforms, and the advocacy never truly ends for the destination keeps shifting. Even when you think you have accomplished your goal, there are always efforts to undermine it, which pushes you away from it, and the journey begins anew.

America's Return on Investment: The Case for Prioritizing Health Equity

The journey to health equity starts from a distant point. According to the National Academy of Medicine, over the past one hundred years, Americans have added thirty years to their life expectancy, but only five of those years are directly attributable to health care. America spends more on health care than any other country on Earth, but it is not the healthiest nation. According to the World Bank, in 2019, the United States ranked forty-third in life expectancy in the world, a troubling ranking given that America consumes more than half of the world's health care resources. Even more alarming, America's life expectancy ranking is expected to drop twenty-one points to sixty-fourth in the world in the next two decades, according to research published by *The Lancet*. In the rest of the world, by contrast, life expectancies are expected to rise by an average of 4.4 years, while the United States will only see a rise of a little over one year.[1] According to Professor Sir Michael Marmot, an internationally renowned scholar on the social determinants of health, "life expectancy as a measure of health tells us a great deal how we are doing as a society, and the inequalities in health tell us even more about a society."[2]

In the 1970s, the gap in life expectancy between lower and higher socioeconomic status communities started significantly narrowing, and both groups, in general, saw their life expectancies increase, a trend similar to that of other industrialized nations. However, starting in the 1980s, the life expectancy gap began to widen, and increases in life expectancy slowed. Today, any gains realized in life expectancy overall in the last century, notwithstanding the slowdown experienced in the 1980s, are quickly disappearing as the United States grapples with an alarming trend not seen since World War I. For several years in a row, the life expectancy rate in the United States has declined owing to a host of factors, including suicides, drug overdoses, obesity, diabetes, cancer, and the rise in heart disease. This crisis has been accompanied by another equally troubling pattern: increases in health disparities combined with regressions in areas where positive health outcomes had been seen across the board for population groups.

When life expectancy is disaggregated by race, the inequities among groups are startling. If white Americans were a country, it would rank 50th in the world. If black Americans were a country, it would rank 103rd in the world. If Native Americans were a country, it would rank 143rd in the world. What if we were all equal in the United States? Looking at health care alone, independent of other factors that impact our health, could help to reduce these disparities, but they would not eliminate these disparities. Dr. David Satcher, the sixteenth US surgeon general and a preeminent health policy expert, writing with other health policy researchers, noted that between 1991 and 2000, more than 176,600 deaths were averted through medical advances, and if we had eliminated racial disparities in health care, approximately 886,200 African American lives would have been saved.[3] Imagine how many more lives would have been saved since 2000 if we successfully addressed not just health care disparities but also disparities in health status and the non–health care determinants that have led to these results. Economically, if we were to eliminate

American racial health disparities, we would save over $300 billion per year. These figures do not include premature deaths or the cost burden owing to disparities in health status affecting people with disabilities, LGBTQ+ individuals, women, veterans, and other vulnerable populations. The seminal question as we move forward is, *How have these inequities continued, and why has the United States, with its advanced health care and economic system, not seen better results?*

More than forty years had passed since the US government held its first-ever congressional hearing to specifically address minority health and health disparities in the country. During the 1979 hearing, policy makers highlighted the diminished quality of care afforded racial and ethnic minorities, the lack of diversity in the health care workforce, and the poor health outcomes among lower socioeconomic status individuals and minorities. After that hearing, Congress charged the Institute of Medicine—now the National Academy of Medicine—to examine the issue further and develop a report titled *Health Care in a Context of Civil Rights*, which highlighted racial, socioeconomic, and disability differences in health care. Forty years later, not much has changed since that report was published. There is still a lot left to do relative to accessibility and diversity of clinical trials, medical curricula, access to care and treatments, delivery of care (including behavioral health services), and the health care workforce. In many respects, we have regressed in some areas. However, health care is but a subset of a larger systemic problem that has produced health disparities. Certainly, progress has been made in understanding the importance of emotional and mental health to systemic health and in integrating emotional and mental health downstream, but we must continue venturing further upstream to tackle the structural barriers in our society that limit success in eliminating disparities and realizing better health outcomes.

One striking point from that 1979 congressional hearing and the ensuing report was the following: "Although a full commitment to equality has never characterized American health policy, ... serious questions arise whether the present partial commitments to equality in healthcare will be maintained."[4] While it is shocking to read the unequivocal acknowledgment that we have never experienced a full commitment to health equality in America, even more concerning is that health equity leaders in 1979 doubted that even the limited gains they had achieved would be maintained into the future. They were right. With our demographic shifts, decreases in life expectancy, and poorer health status, we can no longer afford to embrace a partial commitment to equality in health care or tolerate the dearth of public policies addressing health inequalities.

Moving beyond Merely Nibbling at the Edges: Understanding, Managing, and Leveraging the Political Determinants of Health

Earlier, I mentioned that US citizens had added thirty years to their life expectancy, but only five of those years were attributed to better health care access and higher quality care. The other twenty-five years have been attributed to non-health care factors, including prevention and public health initiatives, affordable housing, education, employment, transportation, and other resources necessary to thrive in a society. Today, researchers have classified these as social determinants of health. According to Dr. Brian Smedley, a nationally distinguished expert, "recent bi-partisan interest in addressing the social determinants of health is an important development that hopefully will correct some of the imbalance in the United States' investments in health—today, less than five cents of every federal health dollar is invested in prevention. But to make progress on some of our most deeply embedded health inequities, including racial, ethnic, and socioeconomic, improving the social determinants of health alone will not assure health equity."[5]

As we dig further into these social determinants to understand their interrelationships and how they have caused health inequities, we now recognize they rest on underlying political determinants undergirded by structural racism and other insidious forms of discrimination. These political determinants must be examined, understood, appropriately managed, and leveraged to address the structures and systems that have prevented the realization of health equity in America. Otherwise, we will continue to "merely nibble around the edges of the problem," as Smedley declares.[6] The United States, along with every other country, must seriously address the political determinants of health or else perpetuate the myth that existing inequities were purely socially derived or that inequities are so far removed from a political determinant that inequities can no longer be linked to a political determinant, thus severing any legal mechanisms to correct them. This will mean engaging in uncomfortable conversations on inequities stemming from race, ethnicity, place, and class; disrupting the fragmentation between systems; forging more thoughtful and effective partnerships; and expending the resources necessary to address these dynamics and achieve health equality.

As I mentioned in chapter 3, the political determinants of health involve the systematic processes of structuring relationships, distributing resources, and administering power, operating simultaneously in ways that mutually reinforce one another to shape opportunities that advance health equity or create, perpetuate, and exacerbate health inequities. These political determinants of health are the instigators of the causes of inequities, the determinants of the determinants, which have a cascading effect on our health and life. Over time, health inequities owing to political action or inaction have become so structurally entrenched that it has been difficult to identify their root causes. The failure to invest the time and resources necessary to understand, manage, and leverage political determinants of health is why it is difficult to stem the tide of inequities and achieve health equality. Fortunately, there have been successes in overturning precedent and setting new precedent; however, it has taken tremendous political will and capital to effect those changes.

A Case Study: Jessica's Story

Let us consider a hypothetical[7] example that combines the experiences of real people in urban and rural communities. It highlights the complex intersections of the political determinants of health model.

Imagine a nineteen-year-old woman (we will call her Jessica) who has had several miscarriages. She finally gives birth to an infant nine weeks early, weighing just three pounds, but Jessica almost dies during delivery. Underdeveloped, her baby is placed in the neonatal intensive care unit and tests done on the baby's umbilical cord blood reveal it contains over two hundred toxins. How and why did these results occur? Where did the system fail Jessica and her baby?

Three years earlier, Jessica had left her parents' house owing to her father's substance use disorder. For ten years prior to that, her dad could access the health services and treatments he needed to remain sober, but then policy makers decided to decrease funding for mental health and substance use services and closed down three of the city's five public community mental health centers to "save" money. When her dad's condition worsened, he ended up in an altercation at work, badly beating a coworker, resulting in his termination and arrest. Her mother, who only received a middle-school education, could not secure a job with a livable wage because she did not have the requisite skills and became depressed. She, like her husband, could not access mental health services because of policy makers' decision to close down three of the five public community mental health centers.

After enduring the trauma of witnessing her parents' decline in mental health and financial hardship and succumbing to stress, Jessica eventually moved to an apartment in a low-income neighborhood. Convenience stores and fast-food restaurants dotted every intersection, sidewalks were scarce, city buses did not run through her community, health care providers refused to operate in the community owing to poor reimbursement rates from Medicaid, and schools were failing. Each of these neighborhood conditions were politically determined. Politicians determined whether to create and keep housing segregation in place and whether to expend resources to build sidewalks, parks, or recreational facilities in the community so individuals could walk, play, and exercise. Politicians had determined whether to create a bus route through the community to other more resourced communities or whether to incentivize grocery stores to operate in the community and provide access to fresh fruits, vegetables, and meat. And even when community members decided to take matters into their own hands to try to establish a community garden and operate a farmer's market, politicians failed to issue a permit allowing them to proceed with the project. Politicians also influenced decisions to cover obstetrical, gynecological, or other health services under government health insurance programs or to increase reimbursement rates to incentivize providers to serve poorer populations.

In her community, county policy makers even changed the zoning laws to permit development of a dump site, a chemical plant, and state policy makers switched the source of their water from a clean river ten miles away to a nearby river that was more polluted because of the chemical plant—again to "save" money. This water was used not only to drink, bathe, and wash clothes but also to irrigate the lawn around her apartment building. Over the years pollutants had seeped into the soil and the air creating additional environmental hazards. Children played on the grass and dug in the dirt, and parents never realized the impact these toxins, like lead, were having on their children's health. Her district lacked tenant rights, and, with no rental inspection program, landlords failed to remediate unhealthy housing.

Jessica found a minimum wage job at one of the convenience stores in her community, which did not provide employee benefits such as health insurance, disability insurance, or contributions to an employee retirement fund. As a result, she was kept in poverty because state policy makers rejected proposals to increase the minimum wage to a livable wage. While the store did not provide a livable wage, it did provide free snacks during her shifts. Not realizing the effect that high-fat, high-sodium foods would have on her or her baby's health, she gladly took advantage of the free snacks to save money. Healthier foods were more expensive, but she had no access to public transportation to get to grocers' or farmers' markets that offered fresh and nutritious foods. Because the city's policy makers had struck down an effort to ban smoking in convenience stores and other establishments, and because Jessica lacked the wherewithal or the skills to quit her job, she felt she had no other choice but to work in the convenience store where smoking was permitted.

Jessica understood the importance of receiving prenatal services and tried to sign up for health insurance coverage, but her non-ACA-compliant plan denied her maternity coverage. She was already pregnant, a preexisting condition. She tried to sign up for Medicaid, the government's health insurance program for low-income families, but was told that she was not poor enough and thus did not qualify. She saved up what little she could and, with the help of a friend who had a credit card and access to a smartphone, used a ride-sharing service to get to a clinician on the other side of town. Fortunately, the city had recently decided to overturn its previous decision to prohibit ride-sharing services, so she was able to take advantage of it. After waiting half the day to be seen, she finally met the clinician who was condescending and offensive. She could not afford to continue to take days off work and never went back.

At thirty-one weeks, Jessica developed gestational (or pregnancy-induced) hypertension and started experiencing severe headaches, nausea, and visual impairment. Luckily, she found a neighbor with a car who drove her to a hospital emergency department twenty miles away. She was diagnosed with preeclampsia and, by this point, was experiencing excessive swelling in her face and ankles as well as seizures. The emergency team decided to deliver her premature son immediately. Afterward, he was sent to the neonatal intensive care unit. Once his organs were deemed mature enough, he was taken off the machines and sent home with severe cognitive deficits.

At home, Jessica never realized that her baby, who was maturing quickly, was exposed to mildew and cockroaches in the apartment, which caused her son to develop respiratory problems, including asthma. When she did become aware of the issue, Jessica asked the landlord to fix the poor conditions, but he refused, telling her to move if she did not like it. As the baby boy grew, the new mom struggled to find early childhood care and access to schools with educational assistance, healthy food options, and other resources needed to thrive. As he continued to develop, he gained weight, becoming obese. Because their community lacked the resources and the local school was unable to provide the individual educational assistance her son needed to reach his full potential, he dropped out of school after entering eighth grade, as his grandmother had, and likely will repeat the cycle of poverty.

The Lessons from Jessica's Story: Understanding When the Political Determinants of Health Are at Play

Jessica's story reveals a pattern of missed opportunities. First, several social determinants impacted Jessica and her child, including the lack of a support system. She had moved out of her parents' house at the age sixteen owing to their mental condition, which affected her emotionally as well. Jessica lacked suitable means of communication, reliable transportation, access to fresh fruits and vegetables, and the financial resources to adequately take care of herself and her baby.

Second, environmental determinants of health were also apparent and played a crucial role in Jessica's and her son's poor health, exemplified in policy makers' decision to allow a dump site and chemical plant near her community and switch the community's water source to a more polluted source. As a result, Jessica had over two hundred toxins in her system that were passed on to her unborn child. Other environmental determinants affected Jessica and her child, including secondhand smoke at her job and mildew and cockroaches in their apartment, resulting in her son's respiratory problems.

Third, health care determinants intersected with social determinants. Jessica could not obtain adequate health insurance coverage and had challenges accessing quality health services. Once she managed to secure an appointment with a clinician and transportation to the health care facility, she found herself in a hostile environment that was not patient-centered or culturally competent. During her encounter with the clinician, she perceived receiving discriminatory treatment. The perception of discrimination is a social determinant of health.[8] Evidence has shown that perceptions of discrimination were reported by individuals of all races, gender, and income levels during interactions with the police, in the workplace (the most frequently reported), and in everyday life.[9] However, researchers have found a strong implicit preference for white Americans over black Americans in general, and this strong implicit preference has even been found among physicians from various racial backgrounds.[10] Other clinicians, including nurses, dentists, pharmacists, physical therapists, occupational therapists, and behavioral health professionals are also not immune from these biases.

Fourth, behavioral health issues were never addressed. Jessica had experienced several previous miscarriages and the stress of caring for a low-birth-weight baby with developmental disabilities. She had experienced the effects of her father's substance use disorder and her mother's mental health, both conditions that she may be genetically predisposed to inherit. Her visit to the clinician for her sole prenatal visit was a missed opportunity to assess her mental state. This would have given the clinician much insight into who Jessica was, what adverse events she had experienced, and her living conditions. She experienced other behavioral health challenges by working in a place that allowed smoking and offered access to free high-calorie, high-fat, and high-sodium snacks. As her son reached school age, she could not find a school with the resources needed to help him reach his full potential. Dropping out of school created additional behavioral health challenges for both of them.

A closer look at Jessica's social and familial history reveals that the community has failed not only Jessica but also her parents and possibly earlier generations of her family. The story shows that epigenetic effects (nongenetic influences on gene expression) can occur because of political factors, and it may take generations to see the benefit or harm. Over time, the negative effects of the political determinants of health are manifested through a phenomenon known as biological weathering, which leads to accelerated aging of telomeres (which are found at both ends of a person's chromosomes) and poor health outcomes in ensuing generations.

This story demonstrates the inconvenient and harsh truth about the impact of social, environmental, behavioral health, health care, and genetic factors on one's health and over generations, and how collectively these factors contribute to our society's health inequities. It shows the compounding effect of political determinants over personal responsibility. No matter how much Jessica tried to act responsibly, structural, institutional, interpersonal, and intrapersonal obstacles hindered her. Beneath Jessica's notice, political determinants were pulling strings that prevented her and her family from achieving their optimal health and full potential.

Political determinants were at play in this story when policy makers decided to cut back on mental health services for her community, refused to mandate coverage of obstetrical and gynecological services, and authorized poor reimbursement rates from Medicaid, causing lack of access to health care. Further disinvestments occurred when policy makers restricted bus routes, kept her community from becoming greener, denied the issue of permits to establish community gardens and operate a farmer's market, zoned a part of her community for a dump site, and changed the water source, thus negatively affecting the built environment. In addition, the political determinants were in play when policy makers failed to raise the minimum wage to a livable wage, to ban smoking from convenience stores, to invest the resources necessary to ensure the education system could meet the needs of all its students, to create or enforce laws that protected tenants living in unhealthy conditions, and to improve the infrastructure of the community, such as building and maintaining sidewalks and recreational facilities. Collectively, these political determinants negatively impacted Jessica, her son, her parents, and the larger community by preventing them from having a fair opportunity to reach their full health potential.

Jessica's story highlights the multiple systemic factors at various levels impacting an individual, family, and community. It also presents a case for seizing the opportunities we have to leverage the political determinants of health. Imagine how different and more promising the ending to this narrative would have been if a number of changes were made. After identifying the determinants exacerbating health inequities and impacting an individual, her family, and community, one should/we should understand the root causes of these determinants. What may appear to be a social or an environmental determinant usually has a political underpinning. Therefore, while we can achieve some progress in reducing inequities by addressing the social, environmental, health care, and other determinants of health, we cannot root out inequities unless the political factors that have fueled these problems are addressed, given that the political determinants of health are fundamental to all of the determinants of health. If we apply the model outlined in this book, we can provide Jessica and her son a happier ending.

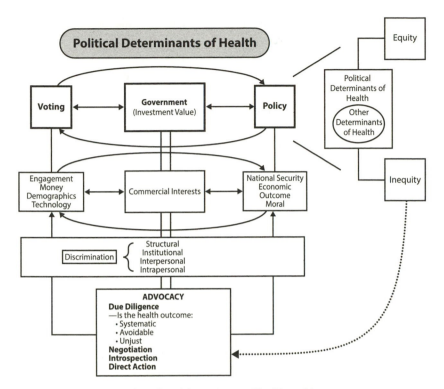

The political determinants of health model.

The Lessons from Jessica's Story: Understanding the Operational Levels of Political Determinants of Health

In Jessica's story, political determinants, both historical and contemporary, at the local, state, and federal levels, truly instigated the challenges and inequities she experienced. It is important to understand when the political determinants of health are at play, on which levels they operate, and who has the jurisdiction to resolve the issue so that an effective advocacy strategy can address the problems. At the local level, policy makers did not provide equal access to public transportation. They approved zoning laws that ensured housing segregation and created difficulties for lower socioeconomic status people to access affordable housing in more resourced communities. Policy makers permitted a dump site and chemical plant in a community that did not have the wherewithal to resist. Policy makers at the local level failed to exercise their authority to promote smoke-free work environments, to provide underresourced schools with critical resources for students' success, to ensure access to safe and affordable housing, or to establish recreational areas in the community as well as community health centers and women's health facilities.

At the state level, policy makers were responsible for redirecting the water source to a more polluted one without first testing and later filtering the water, which led to adverse environmental and health impacts. State-level policy makers rejected multiple attempts to raise the minimum wage and help Jessica attain a livable wage. Further, no policy required that employers provide employee benefits, which caused her to remain in a cycle of poverty.

Although states have the option to expand Medicaid programs, their option resulted from a federal legal decision. The federal government is responsible for the poor reimbursement rates for Medicaid and lack of monitoring of non-ACA-compliant insurance programs. These failures contributed negatively to the issues affecting Jessica and her surrounding community.

Moving from Understanding to Acting: Developing an Advocacy Strategy to Advance Health Equity

After identifying the issues and after fleshing out the underlying political determinants, think about how their resolution would align with current priorities at different levels of power and their probability of success in various advocacy scenarios. This is important because sometimes you may not be able to prioritize issues you deem most important to address if external forces are preoccupied with something they deem more pressing and you are unable to refocus their attention at the time. After weighing the strengths and weaknesses of each scenario, it is time to decide how you will move forward and address the issue or issues you want to resolve.

Identify political champions at all levels (the mayor, commissioners, the governor, legislators, the board of education, the department of transportation, the department of housing, etc.) and determine their effectiveness with regard to elevating or hindering health equity. In addition, identify the commercial interests involved (cellular service and broadband providers, ride-sharing services, hospitals, clinics, credit rating agencies, trade associations, banks, and employers, etc.), as well as the community leaders and affected residents. Even those who may not necessarily be on board or champions for health equity should be consulted because as Elizabeth G. Taylor, executive director of the National Health Law Program reminds health equity proponents, "We are better, stronger and smarter if we are hearing different perspectives."[11] Possible partners to consider in Jessica's case could include (1) environmentalists to address pollution and lack of greenspace/recreation; (2) housing advocates for tenant rights; (3) municipal and state housing authorities; (4) lawyers with particular expertise relative to issues identified; (5) news media to increase awareness; (6) community health workers, including social services and mental health advocates; (7) educational systems at all levels; (8) Planned Parenthood; (9) the local health department; and (10) the local Chamber of Commerce.

Once partners who have agreed to work with you are identified, leverage these partnerships to secure additional data that may be needed to bolster your strategy. Request data from your clinical partners, for instance, to determine whether there is a pattern or trend relative to the issue you are interested in tackling. Suppose you are interested in examining the mental health inequities affecting Jessica's family and want to advocate for increasing access to mental health services. You could look at the last ten years of data for the community to ascertain the impact of the policy decision to close three of the five public community mental health centers by investigating whether there was an increase in admissions related to mental health disorders or increases in workplace or community violence. If you are examining maternal and child health issues, you could collect hospital data to determine whether women in Jessica's area have been having babies prematurely as compared to women in other cities that may not have the same zoning issues and toxic water supply.

To address some of the issues raised in this story, you could request higher reimbursement rates from the federal government for Medicaid to incentivize increased services to low-income populations, petition your state government to cover additional services to address social determinants of health issues, and advocate for your state to raise the eligibility criteria for people like Jessica. You could demonstrate the value of investing in change. Usually, this entails showing how it protects the military and economic system (see chapter 3). In Jessica's case, you could argue that the government should intervene early to make Jessica and her son more financially independent rather than dependent on the government for the rest of their lives, or that helping Jessica's son and other children in the community would allow them to develop the skills needed to serve in the military. In the United States, advocates must understand the disquieting and harsh truth that the political determinants of health inequities have rarely been addressed unless their reduction or elimination served other purposes. Once this is understood, advocates stand a better chance of initiating their health equity agenda and seeing it succeed.

America's Political Tug-of-War to Stamp Out Inequities: Why the Past Is Not Past, and How It Continues to Rear Its Ugly Head

Since the United States was founded, there has been a political tug-of-war to stamp out inequities. Each time advocates made some progress in leveraging the political determinants of health by securing the votes needed to place policy makers who were sensitive to health inequities in the government or by advancing policies that would meaningfully prioritize health equity, opponents succeeded in employing much more effective political strategies and undermining the gains that were made. Indeed, there are lessons to be learned from past advocacy attempts to address inequities and advance health equity. There were short-lived victories, immediately following the Civil War, to uproot structural inequities by establishing federal programs to bolster the social and health needs of newly freed people and poor whites. In addition to addressing these needs, advocates successfully leveraged the political determinants of health to afford individual civil rights protections for disenfranchised groups, including property rights, contractual rights, and equal protection laws; political rights, such as the right to vote or hold public office; and social rights, such as access to public accommodations. With these successes, the United States was well on its way to achieving health equity for all persons.

However, eighteen years after the Civil War, the Supreme Court either put on the brakes or completely dismantled these progressive policies, arguing that eighteen years was sufficient time for an oppressed group of people to catch up to the rest of the population. Today, these lingering and persistent inequities have been baked into our institutions, cemented into the structures of our society, making it hard to identify their genesis. As a result, fallacious arguments have been raised in law as justifications for maintaining the status quo or undermining the rights granted once they led to a perceivable increase in power and privilege for certain groups. Our legal and political systems have recycled poor arguments from one case law, statutory law, or other policy to the next, which have ended up in later laws and policies. One can connect the dots in a straight line from one policy to the next policy to the inequities we have today. The laws of yesterday are modernized today.

Inequities Are Systemic: Just Look at Water

The direct relationship between a political determinant and an inequity today is neatly illustrated by water: a confluence of political determinants through history has magnified both access and avoidance inequities. Since water is the life source for all living things, let us consider its disproportionate impact on people of color and on lower socioeconomic status communities. These communities disproportionately lack modern indoor plumbing, are more likely to be exposed to unsafe tap water, disproportionately experience displacement during flooding, and face a newer phenomenon referred to as climate gentrification[12] owing to climate change. The bottom line is that these communities have a difficult time accessing water when it is clean and safe and a difficult time avoiding water when it is polluted and flooding their homes.

According to the Census Bureau, over 1.6 million people in the United States are without modern indoor plumbing, with black Americans twice as likely as white Americans to live without modern plumbing. The data show that African American communities in the rural South, Latinx communities in the rural Southwest, Native American and Alaska-Native communities, Appalachian communities, and migrant and seasonal farm communities are most affected. In majority-black Lowndes County in Alabama, approximately 80 percent of the community is not connected to the municipal sewer system. On the Navajo reservation, accessing water is no easy feat because approximately 40 percent of the nearly one hundred seventy thousand residents still haul water home in bottles or buckets, often at great expense. In addition, poor white communities in rural Appalachia face waterborne diseases at rates rarely seen in developed nations.[13] Among those who do not lack modern plumbing, many people of color and low-income citizens are intentionally exposed to unsafe tap water, as in Flint, Michigan, or unintentionally exposed, as in Newark, New Jersey, and other communities with aging infrastructures and rusting pipes.

Climate change causes severe flooding and other natural disasters and results in increasing gentrification in some coastal cities. Some people may view these "natural disasters" as social equalizers, but "they have disproportionate impacts on the powerless. People of color, the poor, and the elderly tend to live in less desirable, high risk neighborhoods and so they often feel the effects of storms and floods most heavily."[14] After a natural disaster, these communities are the least likely to benefit from the government's help.

> Disasters are becoming more common in America. In the early and mid-20th century, fewer than 20 percent of U.S. counties experienced a disaster each year. Today, it's about 50 percent. According to the 2018 National Climate Assessment, climate change is already driving more severe droughts, floods and wildfires in the U.S. And those disasters are expensive. The federal government spends billions of dollars annually helping communities rebuild and prevent future damage. But an NPR investigation has found that across the country, white Americans and those with more wealth often receive more federal dollars after a disaster than do minorities and those with less wealth. Federal aid isn't necessarily allocated to those who need it most; it's allocated according to cost-benefit calculations meant to minimize taxpayer risk.[15]

It may seem that the political determinants of health operate in simplistically linear, organized phases, since it is, arguably, a systematic process, but that is not the case. Remember the political determinants of health involve systematic processes of structuring relationships, distributing resources, and administering power, operating simultaneously in ways that mutually reinforce one another to shape opportunities that either advance health equity or exacerbate health inequities. So how do we apply the political determinants of health model in a seemingly confusing complex ecosystem? What if defeat looms, for instance, if, after you have employed successful voting strategies that resulted in the election of your candidate, another arm of the government usurps his or her power?

Applying the Political Determinants of Health in a Complex Ecosystem

Flint, Michigan, provides a perfect example of the impact of structural racism and other forms of inequality on residents and the frustration of employing the political determinants of health to address entrenched issues when multiple political levers push and pull to maintain the status quo. Flint's story highlights how health equity is a continuous struggle for power and resources among competing interests and that advocacy is caught in a complex and dysfunctional political system.

In 2011, the powers of the mayor of Flint, Dayne Walling, a Democrat, were usurped by Governor Rick Snyder, a Republican, who stripped him of his mayoral authority and handed that authority to an appointed budget-slashing emergency manager. Several years earlier another governor had done the same, but the city of Flint fought and lost the state takeover in court, costing it more than $245,000. In 2013, the Flint City Council had recommended switching the source of Flint's water to save money, but before they could conduct a due diligence investigation to determine a new source, a nonelected emergency manager decided with the approval of another nonelected state official to authorize the switch of Flint's water supply to the Flint River until a new pipeline was completed.[16] About one year later, the switch to the Flint River water was official, and residents started receiving tap water from the polluted source. Less than two months before I was scheduled to deliver a speech in Flint, Michigan, on May 5, 2015, at the Genesee County Health Department's Annual Public Health Conference on "Securing Our Future: Protecting the Health of Genesee County Children," the Flint City Council had voted to stop using water from the Flint River, which was contaminated with lead, and reconnect with the Detroit water system.[17] However, once again, a state-appointed emergency manager overruled the local policy makers, stating that it would be "incomprehensible" to stop using that water source.[18]

Despite complaints from residents about the water's yellowish-brown color, foul taste, and odor, policy makers assured them that the water was safe to drink, to bathe in, to clean their homes with, and to water their lawns. This was not true. The water contained high levels of lead, a neurotoxin for which there is no safe level of exposure. The damage had already been done. According to a report by Politico, "Hundreds of children have since been diagnosed with lead poisoning, and a dozen Flint residents died of Legionella[19] from drinking river water."[20] Many of these children today show signs of developmental disabilities and irreversible neurological damage. The long-term effects and the intergenerational trauma have yet to be seen.

I have chosen to end this chapter by highlighting the confluence of political determinants that initiated and intensified the water crisis and the unconscionable inequities in Flint, Michigan. But Flint's story is part of a larger story on the inequities that pervade our society. Unfortunately, this is not the first story to emphasize the enduring linkages between race, place, and class, nor will it be the last. When juxtaposing the political determinants that affect Flint with those impacting America's least healthy place—the Mississippi Delta—we can learn important lessons regarding the connections between power, political engagement, and health equity. In one study that used historical analysis, literature review, and analysis of every law introduced in the Mississippi legislature during the 2017 legislative session, it was found that "legislators from the Delta have comparatively little influence in state-level policy making in Mississippi. This lack of power has deep historical roots but persists today."[21] The study concluded that the power imbalance in Mississippi presents challenges concerning the political process as a mechanism to achieve health equity unless the local community with the greatest need can successfully convince leaders outside the area. The Flint community had to learn and overcome this major lesson for which other less resourced and unhealthy communities across the United States and the world must understand to succeed in addressing their concerns.

As a health policy researcher, I have been deeply troubled by my first and ensuing visits to Flint, where political determinants resulted in one of our nation's most unfortunate and disturbing crises. My friends Tonya French-Turner and E. Yvonne Lewis—both residents of Flint, codirectors of the Healthy Flint Research Coordinating Center Community Core,[22] and longtime leaders in the health equity movement—found themselves staring at their own blatant inequities. They first opened my eyes to the host of problems they were confronting: the inequitable treatment from state government, the difficulty in sounding the alarm, the state's resistance to taking ownership and helping Flint fix this politically created mess.

On November 1, 1977, Vice President Hubert H. Humphrey stated, "The moral test of government is how that government treats those who are in the dawn of life, the children; those who are in the twilight of life, the elderly; and those who are in the shadows of life, the sick, the needy and the handicapped." Certainly, many state and local governments, including the federal government, have failed that test for some groups of its citizens, but Flint is emblematic.

In peeling back the layers to get to the root causes, Flint's story has no shortage of responsible (or guilty) actors. From the governor usurping the mayor's power right after the election and appointing a nonelected official—an "emergency" manager—who was not accountable to the community (not once but four times during this period);[23] to the emergency manager washing his hands of responsibility, stating it was not his duty to find out whether the Flint River was suitable for consumption;[24] to state legislators who passed laws authorizing and subsequently increasing the power of emergency managers even though Michigan voters, through a November 2012 ballot proposal, had repealed the controversial law;[25] and to state policy makers passing and enacting the "second-most stringent local taxation limits in the country, placing 'tremendous pressure on local lawmakers' ability to generate critical revenue,'" there were political determinants operating at various levels that were responsible for this problem.[26] The story, in effect, highlights how one political determinant after another resulted in a continual tightening of a chokehold on Flint and the eventual disaster that brought to light the inequities plaguing it. The story of Flint not only exposes the seriousness of an incompetent government but also reveals an incompetent government that failed to value all of its residents equally and used its power to further relegate them to the most abysmal position.

The resilience of Flint's residents is evident in my interviews; however, many residents seem to have lost hope in the political process. After they elected the mayor, the governor usurped his power. When they initiated grassroots advocacy and convinced the electorate in the 2012 election to pass a citizen-initiated ballot measure to repeal the state's emergency manager law, the governor and state legislators ignored them and passed legislation strengthening the power of a state-appointed emergency manager.

Despite numerous protests by the residents of Flint who toted jugs of the polluted water to community forums, their pleas went unheard. Understandably, residents were also wary of the process when a group of clergy and residents filed a lawsuit against the city, arguing that the river water was a health risk, but the city attorney pushed back, stating that the lawsuit was baseless. The case was dismissed three months later. These failed attempts to address their situation are concerning because if political determinants caused their problems and if political determinants of health are truly the causes of causes—the force that concretized these structural inequities—then communities such as Flint should not give up hope but, instead, continue to use the knowledge of how this system works to effect the necessary changes to help them achieve health equity for all members of their community.

Fortunately, in March 2015, Flint residents continued in their struggle for justice and began to see some hope when one resident contacted the federal Environmental Protection Agency, which then contacted the state environmental agency with data they had collected showing alarming rates of lead in the water. When that did not seem to get the state's attention, the EPA sent a memo to an investigator at the American Civil Liberties Union (ACLU) who shared it publicly through the news media. With data from Virginia Tech researchers showing substantial levels of lead in the water, data from medical researchers showing high lead levels in children's blood, and pressure from the ACLU and the tireless advocacy of residents who employed strategic efforts to recruit champions to help amplify their voices, the state government began to worry about the increased news around Flint's water crisis. The state decided to finally change the source of the water to its original unpolluted source.[27]

One month later, Flint residents filed a federal class action lawsuit claiming that fourteen state and city officials, including Governor Snyder, knowingly exposed Flint residents to toxic water. A month after residents filed a federal class action lawsuit, Flint declared a state of emergency, and the following month the governor felt compelled to declare a state of emergency for Genesee County. By this time, the federal government launched an investigation. With continued advocacy, the residents of Flint, working in concert with the Michigan Civil Rights Commission, convened a series of hearings to examine the causes of this crisis and issued a report: *The Flint Water Crisis: Systemic Racism through the Lens of Flint*, which concluded, "'Deeply embedded institutional, systemic and historical racism' indirectly contributed to the ill-fated decision to tap the Flint River for drinking water as a cost-saving measure."[28] The crisis in Flint not only demonstrates the complexity of the political determinants but also provides us with a plan for action in uncovering, examining, and addressing inequities that plague other communities.[29]

Today's poor health outcomes, lower life expectancy, and health inequities in the United States and in other countries did not happen overnight but was the result of compounding intentional political determinants. For too many countries, the political determinants of health inequities have triumphed over the political determinants of health. In the United States, there has been a tug-of-war between these two competing efforts. And just as we have seen with water, we have seen with food, another basic but critical life source, which has also been subject to political determinations and has led to disturbing inequities among lower socioeconomic status people and people of color.

Inequities Are Systemic: Looking at the Politicization of Another Life Source

Immediately following its founding, the US government rejected arguments that it had a responsibility to ensure proper food and other subsistence to enslaved people and other vulnerable populations. However, after the Civil War, the federal government changed course in 1865 when there was a scarcity of food in the South. It passed legislation to provide food and other necessities to freed black and poor white inhabitants. This program lasted seven years before Congress terminated it. Beginning in the 1930s, the federal government intervened to provide some aid to school boards that were struggling with providing food to their students. During World War II, the federal government recognized a major problem when the military rejected significant numbers of recruits owing to malnutrition. These rejections raised national security concerns, which led to enactment of a narrowly tailored bill, the National School Lunch Act in 1946 and to the federal government inserting itself into school lunch programs.

Then, in 1968, after a "CBS documentary, *Hunger in America*, revealed that too many Americans were suffering from undernutrition," a Senate Select Committee on Nutrition and Human Needs was established, followed by a White House Conference on Food, Nutrition, and Health requested by President Richard Nixon "to explore what policies were required to eliminate poverty-related malnutrition and to enhance nutrition-related health in the United States."[30] The Senate Select Committee would later spearhead the "passage of legislation that vastly expanded food stamp and school lunch programs and introduced the Special Supplemental Nutrition Program for Women, Infants, and Children."[31] In 1971, fearing that the Vietnam War and soaring food costs were threatening his reelection, President Nixon decided to enlist the assistance of a powerful lobbying group to help him lower food costs and transform the way we eat—farmers—which led to a radical change in food policy that would have far-reaching global implications.[32]

The Nixon administration's plan "pushed farmers into a new, industrial scale of production, and into farming one crop in particular: corn. US cattle were fattened by the immense increases in corn production. Burgers became bigger. Fries, fried in corn oil, became fattier. Corn became the engine for the massive surge in the quantities of cheaper food being supplied to American supermarkets: everything from cereals, to biscuits and flour found new uses for corn."[33] Several years later, by the mid-1970s, there was a surplus of corn, and the government looked into other innovative ways to market it. One way was to mass produce high-fructose corn syrup, a very sweet syrup from surplus corn that was relatively cheap to produce. High-fructose corn syrup was

> soon pumped into every conceivable food: pizzas, coleslaw, meat. It provided that "just baked" sheen on bread and cakes, made everything sweeter, and extended shelf life from days to years. A silent revolution of the amount of sugar that was going into our bodies was taking place. In Britain [as well as the United States and other countries], the food on our plates became pure science—each processed milligram tweaked and sweetened for maximum palatability. And the general public [was] clueless that these changes were taking place.[34]

The general public was also clueless about the effect of poor nutrition on their health, but countries started noticing increases in heart disease, diabetes, cancer, and a newer disease, obesity, which was exacerbating heart disease, diabetes, and cancer and, as a result, started to investigate.

According to Dr. Gerald M. Oppenheimer and Dr. I. Daniel Benrubi, "By 1976, the relationship between nutrition and health had become a major preoccupation of the [US Senate Select Committee on Nutrition and Human Needs]; they were particularly interested in 'food additives and health, diet and disease, nutrition research, and the monitoring of nutritional health,'" which was owing to the committee's perception "that millions of American consumers wanted better health information and safer food."[35] As a result, the committee "believed that current government policies were insufficient, and, therefore, 'congressional oversight of nutrition and health' was an 'urgent matter.'"[36] What transpired next was the development and release of a landmark congressional report in the final year of the committee's tenure, named after the chair of the committee, Senator George McGovern, which set off a heated debate among health care and public health experts, commercial interests representing the food industry, and policy makers. Advocates from the food industry decried the lack of consensus among public health professionals regarding the causes of obesity and heart diseases and lobbied to change the language in the report that hurt its interests. The food industry was successful in its lobbying effort, and Congress acquiesced in changing the language in the report and halted its efforts to push back on the industry.

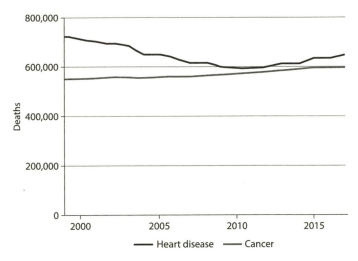

Heart disease and cancer trends in the United States.

Today, the impact from these political determinants regarding food is evident. According to the data, "the number of overweight and obese people worldwide has increased from 857 million in 1980 to 2.1 billion in 2013. Of these, 671 million are obese."[37] By 2030, researchers "project 65 million more obese adults in the USA and 11 million more obese adults in the UK," resulting in "an additional 6-8.5 million cases of diabetes, 5.7-7.3 million cases of heart disease and stroke, 492,000-669,000 additional cases of cancer, and 26-55 million quality-adjusted life years forgone for USA and UK combined."[38] However, like water, food is but one issue in a larger scheme of issues where unequal and unfair distribution impact the most vulnerable. As we layer on the factors affecting health along with the political determinants of health and their interaction with commercial interests, we see a clearer picture of the evolution of inequities and poor health outcomes in our society. By examining the context for each problem, looking at the historical events that have led to the inequities and poor health outcomes in our society and addressing their structural determinants, we stand a better chance of improving the conditions of daily living in struggling communities.

Conclusion: Dispelling Myths, Embracing Truth, and Mobilizing for Bold Action to Realize a Healthy, Equitable, and Inclusive Society

For those who may question whether it is worth the time and effort to address the political determinants of health, Martin Luther King Jr. had this to say in an address at Western Michigan University on December 18, 1963, just four months after delivering his "I Have a Dream" speech:

> Now the other myth that gets around is the idea that legislation cannot really solve the problem and that it has no great role to play in this period of social change because you've got to change the heart and you can't change the heart through legislation. You can't legislate morals. The job must be done through education and religion. Well, there's half-truth involved here. Certainly, if the problem is to be solved then in the final sense, hearts must be changed. Religion and education must play a great role in changing the heart. But we must go on to say that while it may be true that morality cannot be legislated, behavior can be regulated. It may be true that the law cannot change the heart but it can restrain the heartless. It may be true that the law cannot make a man love me but it can keep him from lynching me and I think that is pretty important, also. So there is a need for executive orders. There is a need for judicial decrees. There is a need for civil rights legislation on the local scale within states and on the national scale from the federal government.[39]

Today, the health equity movement is at a tipping point. The United States must decide whether to move forward and embrace a more inclusive, equitable, and healthy society or reverse course, as it has in the past, wiping out any momentum in reducing disparities and exacerbating inequities among population groups. During the advocacy for the Civil Rights Act of 1964, King stated he was "convinced that the people of ill-will in our nation have often used time much more effectively than the people of good will" and voiced his frustration with the stunts that were being employed to delay and prevent the bill's passage. He further stated, "We still see delaying tactics. We still see evasive schemes being used. We still see southern congressmen tying up basic legislation in a particular committee, in this instance, the Rules Committee. We still see the possibility of the filibuster ahead in the senate. There is a great need at this hour for all people of good will of this nation to get together and say that this legislation must be passed and that it must be passed soon."[40] Not surprisingly, advocates for racial equality in 1790, 1864, 1964, and 2010 all had to endure the same political stunts to prevent the passage or implementation of landmark legislation intended to eliminate health disparities and bolster health equity. At the state level, advocates have had to endure additional obstacles to bolster policy priorities. What motivated individuals such as William Lloyd Garrison, Frederick Douglass, Dorothea Dix, W. E. B. Du Bois, Martin Luther King Jr., W. Montague Cobb, Charles Drew, Daniel Inouye, Edward Kennedy, Louis Stokes, Louis Sullivan, Edward Roybal, Daniel Akaka, Donna M. Christensen, Marian Wright Edelman, David Satcher, Georges Benjamin, Michael Bird, Grace Napolitano, Raul Yzaguirre, Elena Ong, and other trailblazers in the health equity movement was an understanding of the power of the political determinants of health to create a healthy, equitable, and inclusive society.

The political determinants of health framework was created to help health equity proponents think more strategically and thoughtfully about the relationship between the political determinants of health and other determinants of health, the intersectionality of commercial and governmental interests, as well as the structural racism and other forms of discrimination undergirding them. Collectively, these determinants of health have over time created, perpetuated, and exacerbated health inequities that have seriously impacted the health of generations of racial and ethnic minorities, Native Americans, Alaska Natives and Native Hawaiians, people with disabilities, women, LGBTQ+ individuals, and those of lower socioeconomic status.

Fortunately, these structural barriers and the resulting inequities are not permanent, but it will take greater action and collective agreement from individuals (Republicans, Democrats, Independents, and others) committed to stomping out inequities to formulate and execute the strategies to overcome them. Before that can happen we must educate ourselves about the history of our communities and understand the political determinants that have driven these inequities in our communities for generations. Only then will we stand a chance of raising consciousness at all levels about these systemic issues and effect meaningful and lasting changes needed to create a healthy and an empowered population. In moving forward with your health equity agenda, it is worth remembering the late Senator Paul Wellstone's words, "Our politics are our deepest form of expression: they mirror our past experiences and reflect our dreams and aspirations for the future."[41] If we want to reflect a healthier, inclusive, and equitable society, then we cannot leave, for future generations, the inevitable task of correcting the political determinants of health inequities that will have even more serious implications for everyone. If we want history to look favorably upon us, then we certainly have a lot of work to do.

Acknowledgments

This new framework, the political determinants of health, is built on years of multidisciplinary research focused on health inequities and the plethora of determinants that have driven these results in our society. It encapsulates the interventions that have been used in the past to advance health equity so that proponents may realize more successes in the future. The ideas, arguments, and conclusions shared in this book resulted from years of collaboration and cooperation with a host of remarkable scholars, researchers, advocates, and leaders whose insights collectively resulted in the final framework.

I want to first thank my family for their unwavering support and help during the writing of this book. To my beautiful wife, Nedeeka, and our children, Raymond and Marc, you are all a blessing to me, and I thank you for your love, encouragement, patience, and understanding while I spent hours researching, traveling for interviews, compiling my thoughts, and writing this book. To my awesome parents, Edward and Mernel, and brothers, Patrick and David, thank you for your never-ending love and support. You all have been my guiding lights, and I thank God for each of you.

Successful completion of any project, especially those designed to bolster health equity, results from teamwork and the collective efforts of a committed community. I am fortunate to work with and learn from some of the most talented and brilliant advocates, scholars, and leaders in health policy.

I want to thank my remarkable editor, Robin W. Coleman, my exceptional copy editor, Andre Barnett, who brilliantly enhanced the quality of this book, and the entire team at Johns Hopkins University Press, who early on recognized the importance, novelty, and authority of this work and provided incredible guidance and support during the writing and publishing process. I will always be grateful to you and your colleagues,

Barbara Kline Pope, Gregory M. Britton, Adelene Jane Medrano, Juliana McCarthy, Heidi M. Vincent, Terrence Melvin, Kathryn Marguy, Tom Broughton-Willett, Rebecca Rozenberg, and others who labored tirelessly to produce and promote this book at JHUP.

I want to specially thank Professors Suzanne Ferriss and Steven Alford for providing me invaluable mentorship, substantive feedback, and tremendous help editing the manuscript. I could never have asked for a better sounding board throughout the writing process. I will always be grateful to you both for taking the time to help me bring these chapters to life as we push the boundaries of our knowledge on this important issue.

I also want to specially thank Professor Catherine Lee Wilson of the University of Nebraska College of Law, who took the time to thoughtfully review the manuscript and provided invaluable information and feedback on the framework and its application. And I want to recognize and thank Deans Anna W. Shavers, Richard E. Moberly, Molly M. Brummond, and Professors Craig M. Lawson and John Snowden at the University of Nebraska College of Law for their mentorship and support before, during, and after the writing of this book. To Richard and Judy Weill, the Honorable Vernon C. R. Daniels, and Professor John Gradwohl and the Honorable Jan Gradwohl, I thank you for being a blessing to me and for mentoring me through the years. You all made it possible for me to engage in this important work to advance health equity for all populations. I will always be grateful to each of you.

I have been fortunate to work with an exceptional group of scholars and leaders to whom I could consistently turn for advice, feedback, and constructive criticism while writing this book. I wish to pay special tribute to my interdisciplinary group of advisors: Professor Christopher R. Banks, Dr. Regina Benjamin, Dr. Dayna Bowen Matthew, Dr. Leonie Brooks, Mr. Scott Bryant-Comstock, Dr. Kathy Cerminara, Dr. Teresa Chapa, Dr. Omar K. Danner, Professor Kelly Dineen, Professor Megan Douglas, Attorney Nelson Dunlap, Dr. Martha L. Elks, Dr. Lynda Frost, Dr. Debra Furr-Holden, Dr. Kisha Holden, Professor Robert Gatter, Dr. Garth Graham, Dr. Regina Greenwood, Dr. Karen Grosby, Dr. Bennie Harris, Dr. Sandra Harris-Hooker, Attorney Keith Henderson, Dr. Mario Hernandez, Dr. Christopher Hulin, Dr. Julie Jacko, Dr. Shaneeta Johnson, Dr. J. Preston Jones, Dr. Thomas LaVeist, Dr. Eleanor Lawrence, Dr. Leandris Liburd, Dr. Ken Martinez, Dr. Octavio Martinez, Dr. Robert M. Mayberry, Dr. William McDade, Professor Martha Moore-Monroy, Dr. Krishnan Narasimhan, Dr. Gary D. Nelson, Professor Elizabeth Pendo, Professor

Carolyn Pointer, Dr. Susan Poser, Professor Desiree Ramirez, Dr. Don Rosenblum, Ms. Charmaine Ruddock, Dr. Francois Sainfort, Professor Amy Sanders, Professor Sallie Sanford, Professor Ana Santos Rutschman, Dr. Elsie Scott, Dr. Taya Scott, Dr. Mona Shah, Dr. Brian Smedley, Dr. Robert Speth, Dr. Beverly Taylor, Attorney Elizabeth Taylor, Dr. Erica Taylor, Dr. Leslie Tworoger, Professor Susan Wald Berkman, Sidney D. Watson, Professor Lindsay F. Wiley, Dr. Stanley Wilson, Ms. Kimberly Wise, Mr. Rick Ybarra, and Professor Ruqaiijah Yearby.

I want to also recognize the exceptional assistance I received from Erika Brown Pringle at Georgetown University Law Center whose attention to details and creative talent helped to enhance the book. To my former students, J. C. Gonzalez and Marie V. Wawa, I will always be grateful to you both for helping me with critical edits to ensure that this book would be completed on time.

Special thanks to Art Collins and Susan Grant whose in-depth knowledge of political determinants helped me to think more critically and led to the development of this new framework. You both have been shining stars in the movement to create and advance health equity.

I wish to thank the following exceptional leaders who have been unyielding in their support of me as I labored day and night for over three years to produce this resource: Ambassador Andrew Young and the entire team at the Andrew J. Young Foundation, Congressman John Lewis, Dr. Louis Sullivan, Dr. David Satcher, Dr. Valerie Montgomery Rice, Dr. Regina Benjamin, Dr. Vivek Murthy, Ms. Stacey Abrams, Congresswoman Donna Christensen, Congresswoman Robin Kelly, Dr. Esther R. Dyer, Congresswoman Allyson Y. Schwartz, Congressman Patrick Kennedy, Congressman Jason Altmire, Dr. Larke Huang, Mr. Thomas W. Dortch Jr., Dr. Britt Weinstock, Dr. Jennifer H. Mieres, Ms. Tasha Cole, Ms. Mia Keeys, Mr. Brandon Webb, Mr. Brandon Garrett, Dr. Gary Puckrein, Ms. Gretchen Wartman, Dr. Niva Lubin-Johnson, Mr. Samuel H. Chupp, Dr. Patrice Harris, Mr. Kermit Payne, Mr. Craig Johnson, Ms. Brenda Kane, Ms. Jennifer Luukkonen, Alex and Fatima Djalo Johnson, Mr. David Johns, Mr. Virgil Miller, Ms. Carla Gullatt, Ms. Sherice Perry, Dr. Millicent Gorham, Ms. Sinsi Hernandez-Cancio, Ms. Susan Dreyfus, Ms. Molly Greenman, Ms. Tracy Wareing Evans, Mr. Milton Little, Father Steven Boes, Ms. Alexandra Cawthorne Gaines, Dr. Arthur Evans, Dr. Joia Crear-Perry, Dr. L. Toni Lewis, Ms. Shavon Arline Bradley, Mr. Anton Gunn, Dr. Aletha Maybank, Ms. Natalie Burke, Dr. Christopher Holliday, Ms. Tonya Lopez, Ms. Jennifer Lubin, Dr. Marjorie Innocent, Mr. Blair

Childs, Mr. Duanne Pearson, Ms. Corinne Colgan, Dr. Steven Ronik, and Dr. Vinita Sauder, Mr. Dale Dirks, Mr. Joshua Lewis, Ms. Denise Britt, Ms. Constance Mack-Andrews, Dr. Tabia Akintobi, Dr. Glenda Wrenn, Dr. Elizabeth Ofili, Dr. John Patrickson, and Drs. Peter and Marlene MacLeish.

This book would not have been a reality without the support and encouragement of the Honorable Calvin Smyre, the Honorable Joy Fitzgerald, Mr. Lawrence V. Jackson, Dr. Claire Pomeroy, Dr. Thomas Malone, Dr. Woodrow W. McWilliams III, Dr. Camille Davis-Williams, Mr. Henry "Hank" Thomas, and Dr. Sylvester McRae. Thank you all for helping me to think more thoughtfully about the points that I raise in this book.

The notion of political determinants of health playing an instrumental role in our life expectancy and health status resulted from years of studying law and policy; developing and implementing public policies at the federal, state, and local levels; visiting and learning from members of many urban and rural communities struggling in our nation to advance health equity to understand the root causes of their problems; and working with an interdisciplinary group of community advocates and researchers to examine and address health inequities. Over the course of conducting research and writing this book, I have met brilliant, resilient, and persevering community leaders who never gave up on their communities and who have fought for decades to ensure that every group, every individual was and is given a fair opportunity to reach their full potential. I want to recognize and thank six of those individuals who not only inspired me but also motivated me to keep pressing forward to produce this meaningful resource for health equity champions: Charmaine Ruddock of Bronx, New York; Kimberly Brown-Williams, Gwendolyn Reese, and Carrie Hepburn of St. Petersburg, Florida; and Tonya French-Turner and E. Yvonne Lewis of Flint, Michigan.

There are certainly others who have been supportive and helpful to me during the development of this book who are not listed, and I hope they know how grateful I am to them. Please forgive this omission and know that it was an inadvertent mistake.

Notes

Foreword
Epigraph: O. Solar and A. Irwin, *A Conceptual Framework for Action on the Social Determinants of Health*, Social Determinants of Health Discussion Paper 2 (Policy and Practice) (Geneva: World Health Organization, 2010).

1. Kennedy, "Day of Affirmation Address."

Chapter 1. The Allegory of the Orchard
Epigraph: "Thomas Jefferson to the Republicans of Washington County, Maryland, 31 March 1809," Founders Online, National Archives, last modified June 13, 2018. Original source: *The Papers of Thomas Jefferson*, Retirement Series, vol. 1, 4 March 1809 to 15 November 1809, ed. J. Jefferson Looney (Princeton, NJ: Princeton University Press, 2004), 98-99.

1. The US Department of Health and Human Services has defined health equity to mean the "attainment of the highest level of health for all people. Achieving health equity requires valuing everyone equally with focused and ongoing societal efforts to address avoidable inequalities, historical and contemporary injustices, and the elimination of health and health care disparities." Beadle and Graham, *National Stakeholder Strategy for Achieving Health Equity*.

2. Williams and Collins, "Racial Residential Segregation."

3. Hartley, "Rural Health Disparities."

4. US Department of Health and Human Services, "Minority Population Profiles."

5. US Department of Health and Human Services, "Healthy People 2020."

6. *Merriam-Webster*, s.v. "distributive justice," accessed July 18, 2019, https://www.merriam-webster.com/dictionary/distributive%20justice.

7. White, *Seeing Patients*.

8. White, *Seeing Patients*.

9. Maron, "Should Prisoners Be Used in Medical Experiments?"

10. Gustavsson and MacEachron, "Research on Foster Children."

11. Aratani, "Secret Use of Census Info." See also Minkel, "Confirmed."

12. World Health Organization's definition of *health*. See https://www.who
.int/about/who-we-are/constitution.

Chapter 2. Setting the Precedent

Epigraph: Thurgood Marshall, "The Bicentennial Speech" (annual seminar of
the San Francisco Patent and Trademark Law Association, Maui, Hawaii. May 6,
1987), http://thurgoodmarshall.com/the-bicentennial-speech/.

1. World Health Organization, "Equity."
2. Friedman, *A History of American Law.*
3. Office of the Historian, "The Declaration of Independence, 1776."
4. Friedman, *A History of American Law,* 154.
5. Friedman, *A History of American Law.*
6. "Benjamin Franklin's Anti-Slavery Petitions to Congress." Petition dated
February 3, 1790, was accompanied by a handwritten cover letter by Benjamin
Franklin dated February 9, 1790.
7. "Benjamin Franklin's Anti-Slavery Petitions to Congress [Philadelphia,
February 3, 1790]."
8. The Senate decided not to act on the petition or formally respond to the
arguments that were raised, but the House decided to refer it to a select committee for further consideration.
9. "Abolition of Slavery."
10. An Act for the Relief of Sick and Disabled Seamen.
11. Friedman, *A History of American Law.*
12. Davis, "There Is No Nobel Prize for Plumbers."
13. Manning, "Tragedy of the Ten-Million-Acre Bill," 44.
14. *The Congressional Globe,* 507; Manning, "Tragedy of the Ten-Million-Acre
Bill," 45–46.
15. Pierce, "Veto Message."
16. Freedmen's Bureau Acts of 1865 and 1866. https://www.senate.gov
/artandhistory/history/common/generic/FreedmensBureau.htm.
17. Matthew, *Just Medicine,* 17.
18. A populist and states' rights southern Democrat from Tennessee,
Johnson had been the only southern senator to remain loyal to the Union and
eventually became vice president under President Lincoln. Lincoln had selected
him for his running mate even though Johnson held strikingly opposite views
on most major policy issues, including the belief that the US Constitution
guaranteed people the right to own slaves.
19. Freedmen's Bureau Acts of 1865 and 1866.
20. "Reuniting the Union."
21. The Editors of Encyclopaedia Britannica, "United States Presidential
Election of 1868."
22. Dawes, *150 Years of ObamaCare,* 24.

23. "Reuniting the Union."

24. "Reuniting the Union."

25. The Editors of Encyclopaedia Britannica, "United States Presidential Election of 1868."

26. US Census Bureau, "Table 1."

27. The Home Owners' Loan Corporation was established in June 1933 to help distressed families avert foreclosures by replacing mortgages that were in or near default with new ones that homeowners could afford. It did so by buying old mortgages from banks—most of which were delighted to trade them in for safe government bonds—and then issuing new loans to homeowners. The HOLC financed itself by borrowing from capital markets and the Treasury.

28. Personal interview with Phyllis Vine, September 27, 2018, in Richmond, Virginia.

29. National Institute of Mental Health Community Services Branch, *Annual Report of Program Activities*, 2.

30. King, "The Rising Tide of Racial Consciousness."

31. *The Negro American*, introduction.

32. Carter, "Presidential Statement."

33. Now the National Academy of Science.

34. LaVeist, Gaskin, and Richard, *Economic Burden of Health Inequalities in the United States*; Waidmann, *Estimating the Cost of Racial and Ethnic Health Disparities*.

35. Mission: Readiness, *Ready, Willing, and Unable to Serve*.

36. Mission: Readiness, *Ready, Willing, and Unable to Serve*.

37. Dawes, *150 Years of ObamaCare*.

38. *Habilitation* has been defined as "the assisting of a child with achieving developmental skills when impairments have caused delaying or blocking of initial acquisition of the skills. Habilitation can include cognitive, social, fine motor, gross motor, or other skills that contribute to mobility, communication, and performance of activities of daily living and enhance quality of life." *Miller-Keane Encyclopedia and Dictionary of Medicine, Nursing, and Allied Health*, 7th ed., s.v. "habilitation," accessed February 12, 2019, https://medical-dictionary .thefreedictionary.com/habilitation.

39. Mackenbach, "Political Determinants of Health."

40. "Healthy People 2020" and draft version of "Healthy People 2030."

Chapter 3. The Political Determinants of Health Model

Epigraph: Ruth Bader Ginsburg, world premiere of documentary *RBG*, Sundance Film Festival, January 20, 2019.

1. See Baciu et al., "The Root Causes of Health Inequity," chap. 3.

2. Collier and Horowitz, *The Kennedys*.

3. Institute of Medicine, "Understanding Health and Its Determinants," chap. 2.

4. Alegría, Pérez, and Williams, "Role of Public Policies."

5. US Commission on Civil Rights, *Health Care Disparities*. See also Schroeder, "We Can Do Better."

6. World Health Organization, "Health Policy."

7. World Health Organization, "What Are the Social Determinants of Health?" Emphasis added.

8. For an excellent article arguing that public health professionals need to become more politically astute, see Kickbusch, "The Political Determinants of Health," 1. She states, "Looking at health through the lens of political determinants means analysing how different power constellations, institutions, processes, interests, and ideological positions affect health within different political systems and cultures and at different levels of governance" (1).

9. According to Professor Johan P. Mackenbach, "States and their legislative and executive agencies (parliaments, governments, ministries, . . .) are examples of political structures." See Mackenbach, "Political Determinants of Health," 2.

10. Mackenbach defines *political processes* to "include elections, lobbying and law-making, and can be characterized by, for example, their levels of democracy." Mackenbach, "Political Determinants of Health," 2.

11. Mackenbach defines *political outputs* to "include the laws, taxes, social security benefits, public services, etc. that will ultimately produce the health and other societal outcomes of interest." See Mackenbach, "Political Determinants of Health," 2.

12. Ansell, *The Death Gap*.

13. Marmot and Allen, "Social Determinants of Health Equity."

14. Laverty et al., "Quantifying the Impact of the Public Health Responsibility Deal."

15. Douglas et al., "Applying a Health Equity Lens." See also Gaskin et al., "The Maryland Health Enterprise Zone Initiative"; and Alegría et al., "Role of Public Policies."

16. Komro et al., "Effect of an Increased Minimum Wage on Infant Mortality."

17. Komro et al., "Effect of an Increased Minimum Wage on Infant Mortality."

18. See Baciu et al., "Root Cause of Health Inequity."

19. "Much public medical care throughout American history has had an 'investment value' to the government." See Goodman-Bacon, "I. Health, Education, and Welfare."

20. US Chamber of Commerce, "About the US Chamber."

21. The only year it fell below number one was in 2000 when it dropped to number two behind the Business Roundtable.

22. Oliver, "Healthcare-Related Lobbying Hits $555M in 2017."

23. For an outstanding argument that makes the case to address the interface of the political and commercial determinants of health, see Kickbusch, "Addressing the Interface."

24. Cohen, "Changing Patterns of Infectious Disease"; see also Blodget, "What Kills Us."

25. Yun, Kessler, and Glickman, "We Need Better Answers."

26. Goodman-Bacon, "I. Health, Education, and Welfare."

27. Bor, "Diverging Life Expectancies." See also Monnat, *Deaths of Despair*.

28. According to the US Census Bureau, "In 2016, among the estimated 18.9 million registered nonvoters in America, the most common reason for not voting was dislike of the candidates or campaign issues (4.7 million registered nonvoters), followed by not being interested in the election (2.9 million), being too busy or having a conflicting schedule (2.7 million), and having an illness or disability (2.2 million)." File, "Characteristics of Voters."

29. DeSilver, "U.S. Trails Most Developed Countries."

30. DeSilver, "U.S. Trails Most Developed Countries."

31. DeSilver, "U.S. Trails Most Developed Countries."

32. File, "Characteristics of Voters."

33. Arthur Collins, interview with the author, March 23, 2018.

34. Lopez, Jaspers, and Martínez-Beltrán, "After Democrats Surged in 2018."

35. Lopez et al., "After Democrats Surged in 2018."

36. Lopez et al., "After Democrats Surged in 2018."

37. "Who Draws the Maps?"

38. "Who Draws the Maps?"

39. Douglas, "Missouri Measure Would Undo Voter-Enacted Redistricting Plan."

40. "Cost of Election."

41. Underhill, "Initiative Process 101."

42. "Healthcare on the Ballot."

43. "Healthcare on the Ballot."

44. Ballotpedia, California Right to Health Initiative, https://ballotpedia.org/California_Right_to_Health_Initiative_(2008).

45. Gergen, "A Candid Conversation with Sandra Day O'Connor."

46. See McLeroy et al., "An Ecological Perspective on Health Promotion Programs."

47. Menand, "Supreme Court Case That Enshrined White Supremacy."

48. Lawrence v. Texas, 539 U.S. 558 (2003).

49. According to Politico, even the most diverse Congress in the history of the United States is a highly educated group: "More than 70 percent of the freshman class went to graduate school. A third of them have law degrees and 15 have MBAs. Seven freshmen earned at least two graduate degrees. Kyrsten Sinema (D-AZ) has four." Jin, "Congress's Incoming Class Is Younger."

50. According to the *New York Times*, "About 5 percent of representatives don't have a bachelor's degree, compared with about two-thirds of Americans 25 and older." Chinoy and Ma, "How Every Member Got to Congress."

51. National Research Council, *Measuring Racial Discrimination*.

52. Jones, "Levels of Racism."

53. See Williams and Collins, "Racial Residential Segregation"; Williams and Mohammed, "Discrimination and Racial Disparities in Health"; and Williams and Mohammed, "Racism and Health."

54. Freeman v. Pitts, 503 U.S. (1992). Emphasis added.

55. Shammas, "Telomeres, Lifestyle, Cancer, and Aging."

56. Aaronson, Hartley, and Mazumder, "Effects of the 1930s HOLC 'Redlining' Maps."

57. Donna M. Christensen, interview with the author, December 30, 2018.

58. The civil rights cases were five cases that were consolidated.

59. According to the Brennan Center for Justice, "Since the ruling, several states previously covered under preclearance moved to restrict voting rights. Since then, many states, including several previously covered by Section 5, has [*sic*] moved to implement restrictive voting measures." See "The Voting Rights Act."

60. Fisher v. University of Texas at Austin, 136 S.Ct. (2016); see also Wygant v. Jackson Board of Education, 476 U.S. 267, 275 (1986); and Richmond v. J.A. Croson, 488 U.S. 469 (1989).

61. Watson, "Ferguson and Beyond"; Yearby, "Sick and Tired of Being Sick and Tired"; and Mullings and Schulz, "Intersectionality and Health."

62. Rothstein, *The Color of Law*.

63. Matthew, *Just Medicine*.

64. Martin Luther King Jr., speech at Western Michigan University, December 18, 1963. Emphasis added.

65. Rothstein, *The Color of Law*.

66. Matthew, *Just Medicine*.

67. World Health Organization, "Health Policy."

68. On March 31, 2014, the US Senate passed the Excellence in Mental Health Act (H.R. 4302) as part of the Protecting Access to Medicare Act, which was signed into law by President Barack Obama on April 1, 2014.

69. King, *Letter from the Birmingham Jail*.

70. Braveman, "Health Disparities and Health Equity." See also World Health Organization, "10 Facts on Health Inequities."

71. Watson, "No Affordable Apartments in California?"

72. Dillon, "California's Housing Supply Law Fails."

73. Dillon, "California's Housing Supply Law Fails."

74. Saloner et al., "The Affordable Care Act."

75. Gan et al., "Impact of the Affordable Care Acts." See also Zerhouni et al., "Effect of Medicaid Expansion."

76. Khatana et al., "Association of Medicaid Expansion with Cardiovascular Mortality."

77. HHS Press Office, "Statement from the Department of Health and Human Services on Texas v. Azar."

78. Dr. Alpha Bryan, interview with the author, August 14, 2018.

79. Walshe and Kreutz, "Bill Clinton Accuses Political Press of 'Blindness.'"

Chapter 4. How the Game Is Played

Epigraph: "The Room Where It Happens," from *Hamilton,* music and lyrics by Lin-Manuel Miranda.

1. Gergen, "A Candid Conversation with Sandra Day O'Connor."

2. Wellstone Way, *Politics the Wellstone Way.*

3. Schaefer and Moffit, "McCain Health Care Plan."

4. *Seizing the New Opportunity for Health Reform* (opening statement of Senator Chuck Grassley).

5. *Seizing the New Opportunity for Health Reform.*

6. *Seizing the New Opportunity for Health Reform* (testimony of Tommy Thompson); emphasis mine.

7. "Ted Kennedy and Health Care Reform."

8. Dwyer, "After a Death Seen on Tape"; Snow and Fantz, "Woman Who Died on Hospital Floor."

9. Kaiser Family Foundation, "Eliminating Racial/Ethnic Disparities in Health Care."

10. Kaiser Family Foundation, "Eliminating Racial/Ethnic Disparities in Health Care." Senators Barack Obama and John McCain were the candidates in this election cycle.

11. "Barack Obama's Plan for a Healthy America."

12. Baucus, "Finance Chairman Baucus Unveils Blueprint."

13. Hilda Solis was nominated by President Obama for the Secretary of Labor cabinet post during December 2008 and was confirmed by the US Senate on February 24, 2009. She became the first Latina cabinet member.

14. Obama, "Remarks by the President at the Annual Conference of the American Medical Association."

15. Seabrook, "Healthcare Overhaul Boosts Pelosi's Clout."

16. Martin, "Obama Calls for Health-Care Reform in 2009."

17. Obama recognized that the American Recovery and Reinvestment Act laid the foundation for health reform and appointed Sebelius and DeParle to his team. Obama, "Remarks by President Obama, HHS Secretary-Designate Kathleen Sebelius."

18. Obama, "Remarks by the President at the Opening of the White House Forum on Health Reform."

19. Cooper et al., *Unclaimed Children Revisited.*

20. Executive Order No. 13507.

21. Newton-Small, "And. Here. They. Go."

22. US Senate Committee on Finance, "Finance Leaders Release Health Care Reform Policy Options."

23. Burris, the only African American senator at the time, had filled President Obama's Senate seat.

24. US Senate Committee on Finance, "Health Care Reform from Conception"; and "Baucus, Grassley Release Policy Options."

25. Obama, "Text of a Letter from the President."

26. Letter from Congressional Black Caucus to Barack Obama, June 5, 2009, in the author's possession.

27. *Addressing Disparities in Health and Healthcare*.

28. Invited speakers included Garth Graham, MD, MPH, deputy assistant secretary for minority health, US Department of Health and Human Services; Louis W. Sullivan, MD, chair of the Sullivan Alliance to Transform the Health Professions, former secretary, US Department of Health and Human Services, and president emeritus, Morehouse School of Medicine; Sally Satel, MD, resident scholar, American Enterprise Institute; Rubens J. Pamies, MD, vice chancellor for academic affairs at the University of Nebraska Medical Center; Peter B. Bach, MD, Memorial Sloan-Kettering Cancer Center, pulmonary and critical care physician, former senior advisor to the administrator of the Centers for Medicare and Medicaid Services; Amitabh Chandra, PhD, professor of public policy, Harvard University Kennedy School of Government; Herman A. Taylor Jr., MD, principal investigator / director, Shirley Professor for the Study of Health Disparities, Jackson Heart Study; Barbara Howard, PhD, principal investigator, Strong Heart Study, Medstar Research Institute; William Lewis, MD, for the American Heart Association's Get with the Guidelines; and Bruce Siegel, MD, codirector, Expecting Success: Excellence in Cardiac Care, of the Robert Wood Johnson Foundation Quality Improvement Collaborative, George Washington University School of Public Health and Health Services.

29. *Health Care Disparities* (testimony of Sally Satel).

30. *Health Care Disparities*.

31. Roybal-Allard, "Congresswoman Lucille Roybal-Allard."

32. Murray and Kane, "Pelosi Vows Passage of Health-Care Overhaul."

33. Kessler, "Sarah Palin."

34. American Medical Association, "AMA Supports H.R. 3200"; Garber, "AMA."

35. The Senate proposal was estimated to cost the federal government $1.6 trillion.

36. From 2003 to 2006, the combined cost of health disparities totaled $1.24 trillion in their country. This report also found that in the same time period, eliminating certain health disparities would have reduced direct health care expenditures by $229.4 billion. LaVeist, Gaskin, and Richard, *Economic Burden of Health Inequalities*.

37. Obama, "President Obama Calls Health Insurance Reform Key to Stronger Economy."

Chapter 5. Winning the Game That Never Ends

Epigraph: Ruth Bader Ginsburg, interview on Al Hayat television, Cairo, Egypt, February 2012.

1. Weir, "Nancy Pelosi Fights for Health Care Reform."

2. Saslow and Rucker, "Ted Kennedy Is Celebrated."

3. Obama, "Remarks by the President to a Joint Session of Congress on Health Care."

4. Pear and Calmes, "Obama Aides Aim to Simplify Health Bills."

5. "From Camp David, Obama Gets a Public Option Earful."

6. US Commission on Civil Rights, *Health Care Challenge.*

7. US Senate Committee on Finance, "Baucus Opening Statement"; and "Health Care Reform from Conception."

8. Stewart, "Bachmann."

9. Waidmann, *Estimating the Cost of Racial and Ethnic Health Disparities*; LaVeist, Gaskin, and Richard, *Economic Burden of Health Inequalities.*

10. *Joint Hearing on Eliminating the Social Security Disability Backlog* (testimony of Peggy Hathaway).

11. Affordable Health Care for America Act, "Final Vote for Roll Call 887," http://clerk.house.gov/evs/2009/roll887.xml.

12. US Const. art. I, § 7, cl. 1.

13. Shaw, "Senate Passes Historic Bill"; Reid, "Historic Health Reform Vote."

14. Cohn, "How They Did It"; "Nelson for the Senate."

15. US Senate roll call votes, 111th Cong., 1st sess.; Obama, "Remarks by the President on Senate Passage of Health Insurance Reform"; Pear, "Senate Passes Health Care Overhaul on Party-Line Vote."

16. Lovley, "Harry Reid."

17. Johnson, "AARP, AMA Announce Support for Health Care Bill."

18. John Lewis, interview with the author, September 15, 2014.

19. Winerman, "House Votes Cap Day of Debate on Health Reform."

20. Patient Protection and Affordable Care Act, "Final Vote Results for Roll Call 165."

21. Obama and Biden, "Remarks by the President and Vice President."

22. Department of Health and Human Services, *HHS Action Plan to Reduce Racial and Ethnic Health Disparities.*

Chapter 6. Growing Pains

Epigraph: John F. Kennedy (speech given at Rice University on September 12, 1962), National Archives, https://jfk.blogs.archives.gov/2017/09/12/we-choose-to-go-to-the-moon-the-55th-anniversary-of-the-rice-university-speech/.

1. Plott, "Eric Cantor."
2. Congressional Budget Office, "American Healthcare Act Cost Estimate."
3. Rogin, "States Won by Trump."
4. Kliff, "Obamacare Is Getting More Popular."
5. Taylor, "Trump, McConnell Point Fingers."

Chapter 7. The Future of Health Equity Begins and Ends with the Political Determinants of Health

Epigraph: James Baldwin, *Nobody Knows My Name: More Notes of a Native Son* (New York: Dial Press, 1961).

1. Solly, "United States Drops 21 Spots."
2. Marmot, "Health Equity in England."
3. Satcher et al., "What If We Were Equal?" See also Woolf et al., "Health Impact of Resolving Racial Disparities."
4. Institute of Medicine, *Health Care in a Context of Civil Rights*, 2.
5. Brian Smedley, interview with the author, March 3, 2019.
6. Smedley interview.
7. Jessica's story draws from actual events that have happened across the United States, including events in Genesee County (Flint, MI), Cook County (Chicago, IL), Fulton County (Atlanta, GA); and Senterfitt et al., *How Social and Economic Factors Affect Health*, "One Path," scenario on p. 2.
8. In a national study conducted by National Public Radio, the Robert Wood Johnson Foundation, and the Harvard T.H. Chan School of Public Health, perceptions of discrimination were reported by individuals of all races, genders, and income levels during interactions with the police, in the workplace (the most frequently reported), and in everyday life. Harvard T.H. Chan School of Public Health, Robert Wood Johnson Foundation, and National Public Radio, "Discrimination in America."
9. T.H. Chan School of Public Health et al., "Discrimination in America."
10. Matthew, *Just Medicine*; White and Chanoff, *Seeing Patients*.
11. Elizabeth G. Taylor, interview with the author, January 25, 2019.
12. Harris, "Climate Gentrification."
Climate gentrification occurs when higher-elevated poorer communities have to move when lower-elevated richer communities find their homes are flooding. In low-lying areas of Miami, for example, these communities are expected to see anywhere from fourteen to thirty-four inches of sea rise by 2060, and, as a result, developers see the scarce higher-elevated land areas, which are occupied mostly by low-income communities of color, as a safe investment.
13. McGraw, "Lack of Access to Water."
14. Klein and Zellmer, "Unnatural Disasters and Environmental Injustice."
15. Hersher and Benincasa, "How Federal Disaster Money Favors the Rich."

16. Fonger, "Former Flint EM."

17. On January 12, 2015, the Detroit Water and Sewerage Department offers to reconnect the city with Lake Huron water, waiving a $4 million fee to restore service. However, municipal policy makers declined, citing concerns that water rates could go up more than $12 million each year, even with the reconnection fee waiver. https://www.cnn.com/2016/03/04/us/flint-water-crisis-fast-facts /index.html.

18. CNN Library, "Flint Water Crisis Fast Facts."

19. According to the Centers for Disease Control and Prevention, "Legionella is a type of bacterium found naturally in freshwater environments, like lakes and streams. It can become a health concern when it grows and spreads in human-made building water systems like showerheads and sink faucets." It may lead to Legionnaires' disease, which according to the CDC, "is very similar to other types of pneumonia (lung infection), with symptoms that include: Cough, Shortness of breath, Fever, Muscle aches, Headaches" as well as "other symptoms such as diarrhea, nausea, and confusion." CDC, "Legionnaries' Disease."

20. McClelland, "Dayne Walling Set Off the Flint Water Crisis."

21. Jones, "Political Participation in the Least Healthy Place."

22. Healthy Flint Coordinating Center is a partnership among the University of Michigan–Flint, University of Michigan, and Michigan State University. HFCC is focused on coordinating research conducted in Flint, minimizing duplication of efforts across local universities, elevating the community's voice in the face of academic and government mistrust, and ensuring ethical research is conducted. The aim is to give power and voice to the community, while fully engaging academic research partners in developing and advancing a community-driven research agenda. "Our History."

23. Flint had a total of four emergency managers from November 2011 to April 2015: Ed Kurtz, Mike Brown, Darnell Earley, and Gerald Ambrose. Goodin-Smith, "Flint's History of Emergency Management."

24. Fonger, "Former Flint EM."

25. Michigan's emergency manager law later faced scrutiny in federal court, when plaintiffs argued that the law was unconstitutional because it disproportionately targeted African American communities and continues a "'narrative of structural and strategic racism.'" Goodin-Smith, "Flint's History of Emergency Management."

26. In addition to initiating stringent laws preventing cities from collecting tax revenue to sustain their operations, Michigan's economic fortunes began declining in the early 2000s, resulting in the state diverting revenue-sharing money earmarked for cities to cover its own budget shortfalls. Flint lost out on $54 million. Detroit lost $200 million, contributing to its 2013 bankruptcy, and the subsequent appointment of its own emergency manager. See McClelland,

"Dayne Walling Set Off the Flint Water Crisis"; and Goodin-Smith, "Flint's History of Emergency Management."

27. McClelland, "Dayne Walling Set Off the Flint Water Crisis."

28. CNN Library, "Flint Water Crisis Fast Facts."

29. Michigan Civil Rights Commission, *The Flint Water Crisis*.

30. Oppenheimer and Benrubi, "McGovern's Senate Select Committee," 61.

31. Oppenheimer and Benrubi, "McGovern's Senate Select Committee," 60.

32. Peretti, "Why Our Food Is Making Us Fat."

33. Peretti, "Why Our Food Is Making Us Fat."

34. Peretti, "Why Our Food Is Making Us Fat."

35. Oppenheimer and Benrubi, "McGovern's Senate Select Committee."

36. Oppenheimer and Benrubi, "McGovern's Senate Select Committee."

37. Whiteman, "Worldwide Obesity Rates Increase."

38. Wang et al., "Health and Economic Burden," 815. See also McKay, "Heart Attack at 49."

39. King, "MLK at Western."

40. King, "MLK at Western."

41. Wellstone, "Paul Wellstone Quotes."

Bibliography

Foreword

Kennedy, R. F. (1996). "Day of Affirmation Address, University of Capetown, Capetown, South Africa, June 6, 1996." https://www.jfklibrary.org/learn /about-jfk/the-kennedy-family/robert-f-kennedy/robert-f-kennedy-speeches /day-of-affirmation-address-university-of-capetown-capetown-south-africa -june-6-1966.

Chapter 1. The Allegory of the Orchard

Aratani, L. (2018). "Secret Use of Census Info Helped Send Japanese Americans to Internment Camps in WWII." *Washington Post*, April 6. https://www .washingtonpost.com/news/retropolis/wp/2018/04/03/secret-use-of-census -info-helped-send-japanese-americans-to-internment-camps-in-wwii/?utm _term=.b42220f81687.

Beadle, M. R., and G. N. Graham. (2018). *National Stakeholder Strategy for Achieving Health Equity*. Washington, DC: Department of Health and Human Services, Office of Minority Health. https://minorityhealth.hhs.gov/npa/files /Plans/NSS/CompleteNSS.pdf.

Gustavsson, N. S., and A. E. MacEachron. (2007). "Research on Foster Children: A Role for Social Work." *Social Work*, 52(1), 85–87. doi:10.1093/sw/52.1.85.

Hartley, D. (2004). "Rural Health Disparities, Population Health, and Rural Culture." *American Journal of Public Health*, 94(10), 1675–1678. doi:10.2105/ajph .94.10.1675.

Maron, D. F. (2014). "Should Prisoners Be Used in Medical Experiments?" *Scientific American*, July 2. https://www.scientificamerican.com/article /should-prisoners-be-used-in-medical-experiments/.

Minkel, J. (2007). "Confirmed: The U.S. Census Bureau Gave Up Names of Japanese-Americans in WW II." *Scientific American*, March 30. https://www .scientificamerican.com/article/confirmed-the-us-census-b/.

US Department of Health and Human Services. (2014). "Healthy People 2020." https://www.healthypeople.gov/.

US Department of Health and Human Services. (2018). "Minority Population Profiles." OMH. https://minorityhealth.hhs.gov/omh/browse.aspx?lvl=2&lvlid=26.

White, A. A., III, with D. Chanoff. (2011). *Seeing Patients: Unconscious Bias in Health Care.* Cambridge, MA: Harvard University Press.

Chapter 2. Setting the Precedent

"Abolition of Slavery." (1790). *Congressional Record,* March 5, 1790, 1st Congress, 2nd Session No. 13 (communicated to the US House of Representatives).

An Act for the Relief of Sick and Disabled Seamen. (1798). Stat. 5th Cong., 2d Sess. Library of Congress. http://memory.loc.gov/cgi-bin/ampage?collId=llsl&fileName=001/llsl001.db&recNum=728.

"Benjamin Franklin's Anti-Slavery Petitions to Congress [Philadelphia, February 3, 1790]." (1790). The Center for Legislative Archives, National Archives. https://www.archives.gov/legislative/features/franklin.

Bill for the Benefit of the Indigent Insane. (1851). *The Congressional Globe.* 31st Cong., 2d Sess., February 11.

Carter, J. (1980). "Presidential Statement: Carter Proposes Mental Health Systems Act." In *CQ Almanac* 1979, 35th ed., 31-E-32-E. Washington, DC: Congressional Quarterly. http://library.cqpress.com/cqalmanac/cqal79-861-26160-1182855.

Davis, K. (2018). "There Is No Nobel Prize for Plumbers." Keynote presented at the College for Behavioral Health Leadership: Summit 2018. Virginia Union University, Richmond, September 26–27. https://www.leaders4health.org/summit.

Dawes, D. E. (2018). *150 Years of ObamaCare.* Baltimore: Johns Hopkins University Press.

The Editors of Encyclopaedia Britannica. (2018). "United States Presidential Election of 1868." *Encyclopædia Britannica.* https://www.britannica.com/event/United-States-presidential-election-of-1868.

Friedman, L. M. (2005). *A History of American Law.* 3rd ed. New York: Simon & Schuster.

King, M. L., Jr. (1960). "The Rising Tide of Racial Consciousness." Address at the Golden Anniversary Conference of the National Urban League, New York, New York, September 6, 1960. https://kinginstitute.stanford.edu/king-papers/documents/rising-tide-racial-consciousness-address-golden-anniversary-conference.

LaVeist, T., D. Gaskin, and P. Richard. (2009). *The Economic Burden of Health Inequalities in the United States.* Washington, DC: Joint Center for Political and Economic Studies.

Mackenbach, J. (2014). "Political Determinants of Health." *European Journal of Public Health,* 24(1), 2. https://doi.org/10.1093/eurpub/ckt183.

Manning, S. W. (1962). "The Tragedy of the Ten-Million-Acre Bill." *Social Service Review*, 36(1), 44–50.

Matthew, D. (2015). *Just Medicine: A Cure for Racial Inequality in American Health Care*. New York: New York University Press.

Mission: Readiness. (2009). *Ready, Willing, and Unable to Serve*. Washington, DC: Mission: Readiness. http://cdn.missionreadiness.org/NATEE1109.pdf.

National Institute of Mental Health Community Services Branch. (1957). *Annual Report of Program Activities: January 1, 1957–December 31, 1957*. https://archive.org/stream/reportofprograma1957nati/reportofprograma1957nati_djvu.txt.

The Negro American. (1961). Washington, DC: US Information Agency Office of Research and Analysis.

Office of the Historian. (n.d.). "The Declaration of Independence, 1776." Milestones: 1776–1783. US Department of State. https://history.state.gov/milestones/1776-1783/declaration.

Pierce, Franklin. (n.d.). "Veto Message," May 3, 1854. Online by Gerhard Peters and John T. Woolley, The American Presidency Project. http://www.presidency.ucsb.edu/ws/?pid=67850.

"Reuniting the Union: A Chronology." (2019). Digital History. http://www.digitalhistory.uh.edu/disp_textbook.cfm?smtID=2&psid=3096.

US Census Bureau. (1870). "Table 1. Population of the United States (By States and Territories) in the Aggregate, and as White, Colored, Free Colored, Slave, Chinese, and Indian at Each Census." In *Population by States and Territories—1790-1870*. https://www2.census.gov/library/publications/decennial/1870/population/1870a-04.pdf#.

US Congress House Select Committee on Freedmen. (1865). *Message from the President of the United States, Transmitting Report of the Commissioner of the Bureau of Refugees, Freedmen, and Abandoned Lands*. Washington, DC: s.n.

US Department of Health and Human Services. (2014). "Healthy People 2020." https://www.healthypeople.gov/.

Waidmann, T. (2009). *Estimating the Cost of Racial and Ethnic Health Disparities*. Washington, DC: Urban Institute.

World Health Organization. (2011). "Equity." https://www.who.int/healthsystems/topics/equity/en/.

Chapter 3. The Political Determinants of Health Model

Aaronson, D., D. Hartley, and B. Mazumder. (2017). "The Effects of the 1930s HOLC 'Redlining' Maps." Working Paper Series WP-2017-12, Federal Reserve Bank of Chicago. https://ideas.repec.org/p/fip/fedhwp/wp-2017-12.html.

Alegría, M., D. J. Pérez, and S. Williams. (2003). "The Role of Public Policies in Reducing Mental Health Status Disparities for People of Color." *Health Affairs*, 22(5), 51–64. https://doi.org/10.1377/hlthaff.22.5.51.

Ansell, D. A. (2017). *The Death Gap: How Inequality Kills.* Chicago: University of Chicago Press.

Baciu, A., Y. Negussie, and A. Geller; National Academies of Sciences, Engineering, and Medicine, et al., eds. (2017). "The Root Causes of Health Inequity." In *Communities in Action: Pathways to Health Equity.* Washington, DC: National Academies Press.

Blodget, H. (2012). "What Kills Us: The Leading Causes of Death from 1900–2010." *Business Insider,* June 24. https://www.businessinsider.com/leading-causes-of-death-from-1900-2010-2012-6.

Bor, J. (2017). "Diverging Life Expectancies and Voting Patterns in the 2016 US Presidential Election." *American Journal of Public Health,* 107(10), 1560–1562. https://www.ncbi.nlm.nih.gov/pubmed/28817322.

Braveman, P. (2006). "Health Disparities and Health Equity: Concepts and Measurement." *Annual Review of Public Health,* 27, 167–194.

Chinoy, S., and J. Ma. (2019). "How Every Member Got to Congress." *New York Times,* January 26. https://www.nytimes.com/interactive/2019/01/26/opinion/sunday/paths-to-congress.html.

Cohen, M. L. (2000). Changing Patterns of Infectious Disease. *Nature (London),* 406(6797), 762–767. http://pascal-francis.inist.fr/vibad/index.php?action=search&terms=1498033.

Collier, P., and D. Horowitz. (2002). *The Kennedys: An American Drama.* San Francisco: Encounter Books.

"Cost of Election." (n.d.). OpenSecret.org. https://www.opensecrets.org/overview/cost.php.

DeSilver, D. (2018). "U.S. Trails Most Developed Countries in Voter Turnout." Pew Research Center. https://www.pewresearch.org/fact-tank/2018/05/21/u-s-voter-turnout-trails-most-developed-countries/.

Dillon, L. (2019). "California's Housing Supply Law Fails to Spur Enough Construction, Study Says." *Los Angeles Times,* February 28. https://www.latimes.com/politics/la-pol-ca-housing-supply-law-failures-study-20190228-story.html?hootPostID=fc0fa82db18fe45f83d12e6bb6b388af.

Douglas, C. (2019). "Missouri Measure Would Undo Voter-Enacted Redistricting Plan." KHQA, April 25. https://khqa.com/news/local/missouri-measure-would-undo-voter-enacted-redistricting-plan-04-25-2019.

Douglas, M., R. J. Willock, E. Respress, L. Rollins, D. Tabor, H. J. Heiman, J. Hopkins, D. E. Dawes, and K. B. Holden. (2019). "Applying a Health Equity Lens to Evaluate and Inform Policy." *Ethnicity & Disease,* 29(Suppl. 2), 329–342. doi:10.18865/ed.29.S2.329.

File, T. (2018). "Characteristics of Voters in the Presidential Election of 2016." In *Current Population Reports.* Washington, DC: Census Bureau. https://www.census.gov/content/dam/Census/library/publications/2018/demo/P20-582.pdf.

Gan, T., H. F. Sinner, S. C. Walling, Q. Chen, B. Huang, T. C. Tucker, J. A. Patel, et al. (2019). "Impact of the Affordable Care Act on Colorectal Cancer Screening, Incidence, and Survival in Kentucky." *Journal of the American College of Surgeons*, 228(4), 342–353.e1. https://doi.org/10.1016/j.jamcollsurg .2018.12.035.

Gaskin, D. J., R. Vazin, R. McCleary, and R. J. Thorpe. (2018). "The Maryland Health Enterprise Zone Initiative Reduced Hospital Cost and Utilization in Underserved Communities." *Health Affairs*, October. https://doi.org/10.1377 /hlthaff.2018.0642.

Gergen, D. (2012). "A Candid Conversation with Sandra Day O'Connor: 'I Can Still Make a Difference.'" *Parade*, September 30. https://parade.com/125604 /davidgergen/30-sandra-day-oconnor-i-can-make-a-difference/.

Goodman-Bacon, A. (2016). "I. Health, Education, and Welfare." Review of *150 Years of ObamaCare*, by Daniel E. Dawes. *Journal of Economic Literature*, 54(4), 1401–1402. https://pubs.aeaweb.org/doi/pdfplus/10.1257/jel.54.4.1390.

"Healthcare on the Ballot." (n.d.). Ballotpedia. https://ballotpedia.org/Healthcare _on_the_ballot#By_year.

HHS Press Office. (2018). "Statement from the Department of Health and Human Services on Texas v. Azar." Press release. HHS.gov, December 17. https:// www.hhs.gov/about/news/2018/12/17/statement-from-the-department-of -health-and-human-services-on-texas-v-azar.html.

Institute of Medicine; Durch, J. S., L. A. Bailey, and M. A. Stoto, eds. (1997). "Understanding Health and Its Determinants." In *Improving Health in the Community: A Role for Performance Monitoring*. Washington, DC: National Academies Press. www.nap.edu/openbook/0309055342/html/40.html.

Jin, B. (2018). "Congress's Incoming Class Is Younger, Bluer, and More Diverse Than Ever. *Politico*, November 23. https://www.politico.com/interactives /2018/interactive_116th-congress-freshman-younger-bluer-diverse/.

Jones, C. P. (2000). "Levels of Racism: A Theoretic Framework and a Gardener's Tale." *American Journal of Public Health*, 90(8), 1212–1215.

Khatana, S. A. M., A. Bhatla, A. S. Nathan, J. Giri, C. Shen, D. S. Kazi, R. W. Yeh, and P. W. Groenevelds. (2019). "Association of Medicaid Expansion with Cardiovascular Mortality: A Quasi-experimental Analysis." Abstract 3. *Circulation: Cardiovascular Quality and Outcomes*, 12(Suppl. 1). https://doi.org /10.1161/hcq.12.suppl_1.3.

Kickbusch, I. (2012). Addressing the Interface of the Political and Commercial Determinants of Health. *Health Promotion International*, 27(4), 427–428. doi:10.1093/heapro/das057.

Kickbusch, I. (2015). "The Political Determinants of Health—10 Years On" [Editorial]. *BMJ*, 350:h81.

King, M. L., Jr. (1963). "MLK at Western." Dr. Martin Luther King Jr. 1963 Speech Found. Western Michigan University Archives and Regional History

Collections and University Libraries. https://wmich.edu/sites/default/files/attachments/MLK.pdf.

King, M. L. (1994). *Letter from the Birmingham Jail*. San Francisco: HarperSan Francisco.

Komro, K. A., M. D. Livingston, S. Markowitz, and A. C. Wagenaar. (2016). "The Effect of an Increased Minimum Wage on Infant Mortality and Birth Weight." *American Journal of Public Health*, 106(8), 1514–1516. https://doi.org/10.2105/AJPH.2016.303268.

Krogstad, J. M., and M. H. Lopez. (2017). "Black Voter Turnout Fell in 2016, Even as a Record Number of Americans Cast Ballots." Pew Research Center, May 12. https://www.pewresearch.org/fact-tank/2017/05/12/black-voter-turnout-fell-in-2016-even-as-a-record-number-of-americans-cast-ballots/.

Laverty, A. A., C. Kypridemos, P. Seferidi, E. P. Vamos, J. Pearson-Stuttard, B. Collins, S. Capewell, et al. (2019). "Quantifying the Impact of the Public Health Responsibility Deal on Salt Intake, Cardiovascular Disease and Gastric Cancer Burdens: Interrupted Time Series and Microsimulation Study. *Journal of Epidemiology & Community Health*, 73, 881–887.

Lopez, A., B. Jaspers, and S. Martínez-Beltrán. (2019). "After Democrats Surged in 2018, Republican-Run States Eye New Curbs on Voting." NPR, April 22. https://www.npr.org/2019/04/22/714950127/after-democrats-surged-in-2018-republican-run-states-eye-new-curbs-on-voting.

Mackenbach, J. P. "Political Determinants of Health." *European Journal of Public Health*, 24(1), 2. https://doi.org/10.1093/eurpub/ckt183.

Marmot, M., and J. J. Allen. (2014). "Social Determinants of Health Equity." *American Journal of Public Health*, 104, S517–S519. https://doi.org/10.2105/AJPH.2014.302200.

Matthew, D. B. (2015). *Just Medicine: A Cure for Racial Inequality in American Health Care*. New York: New York University Press.

McLeroy, K. R., D. Bibeau, A. Steckler, and K. Glanz. (1988). "An Ecological Perspective on Health Promotion Programs." *Health Education Quarterly*, 15, 351–377.

Menand, L. (2019). "The Supreme Court Case That Enshrined White Supremacy in Law: How *Plessy v. Ferguson* Shaped the History of Racial Discrimination in America." *New Yorker*, January 28. https://www.newyorker.com/magazine/2019/02/04/the-supreme-court-case-that-enshrined-white-supremacy-in-law.

Monnat, S. M. (2016). *Deaths of Despair and Support for Trump in the 2016 Presidential Election*. Research Brief. University Park: The Pennsylvania State University. https://aese.psu.edu/directory/smm67/Election16.pdf.

Mullings, L., and A. J. Schulz. (2006). "Intersectionality and Health: An Introduction." In A. J. Schulz and L. Mullings, eds., *Gender, Race, Class, & Health: Intersectional Approaches*. San Francisco: Jossey-Bass.

National Research Council. (2004). *Measuring Racial Discrimination*. Washington, DC: National Academies Press. https://doi.org/10.17226/10887.

Oliver, E. (2018). "Healthcare-Related Lobbying Hits $555M in 2017—6 Statistics on Lobbying in Healthcare." *Becker's ASC Review*, January 31. https://www.beckersasc.com/asc-coding-billing-and-collections/healthcare-related-lobbying-hits-555m-in-2017-6-statistics-on-lobbying-in-healthcare.html.

Rothstein, R. (2017). *The Color of Law: A Forgotten History of How Our Government Segregated America*. New York: Liveright.

Saloner, B., R. Landis, B. D. Stein, and C. L. Barry. (2019). "The Affordable Care Act in the Heart of the Opioid Crisis: Evidence from West Virginia." *Health Affairs*, 38(4), 633–642. https://doi.org/10.1377/hlthaff.2018.05049.

Schroeder, S. A. "We Can Do Better—Improving the Health of the American People." *New England Journal of Medicine*, 357, 1221-1228.

Shammas, M. A. (2011). "Telomeres, Lifestyle, Cancer, and Aging." *Current Opinion in Clinical Nutrition and Metabolic Care*, 14(1), 28–34. doi:10.1097/MCO.0b013e32834121b1.

Underhill, W. (2019). "Initiative Process 101." NCSL. http://www.ncsl.org/research/elections-and-campaigns/initiative-process-101.aspx.

US Chamber of Commerce. (2019). "About the U.S. Chamber," March 22. https://www.uschamber.com/about/about-the-us-chamber.

US Commission on Civil Rights. (2010). *Health Care Disparities: A Briefing before the United States Commission on Civil Rights*. Washington, DC: Commission on Civil Rights. https://www.usccr.gov/pubs/docs/Healthcare-Disparities.pdf.

"The Voting Rights Act." (n.d.). Brennan Center for Justice. https://www.brennancenter.org/issues/the-voting-rights-act.

Walshe, S., and L. Kreutz. (2014). "Bill Clinton Accuses Political Press of 'Blindness.'" *ABC News*, April 30. https://abcnews.go.com/blogs/politics/2014/04/bill-clinton-accuses-political-press-of-blindness/.

Watson, L. (2019). "No Affordable Apartments in California? Check Back in a Couple Thousand Years." Splinter, February 28. https://splinternews.com/no-affordable-apartments-in-california-check-back-in-a-1832958684.

Watson, S. D. (2017). "Lessons from Ferguson and Beyond: Bias, Health, and Justice." *Minnesota Journal of Law, Science & Technology*, 18, 111-142.

"Who Draws the Maps? Legislative and Congressional Redistricting." (2019). Brennan Center for Justice. https://www.brennancenter.org/analysis/who-draws-maps-states-redrawing-congressional-and-state-district-lines.

Williams, D. R., and C. Collins. (2001). "Racial Residential Segregation: A Fundamental Cause of Racial Disparities in Health." *Public Health Reports*, 116(5), 404-416. https://doi.org/10.1093/phr/116.5.404.

Williams, D. R., and S. A. Mohammed. (2009). "Discrimination and Racial Disparities in Health: Evidence and Needed Research." *Journal of Behavioral Medicine*, 32, 20-47.

——. (2013). "Racism and Health: I. Pathways and Scientific Evidence." *American Behavioral Scientist*, 57(8), 1152-1173. https://doi.org/10.1177 /0002764213487340.

World Health Organization. (2011). "10 Facts on Health Inequities and Their Causes." http://www.who.int/features/factfiles/health_inequities/en.

——. (2013). "Health Policy." https://www.who.int/topics/health_policy/en/.

——. (2019). "What Are the Social Determinants of Health?" https://www.who .int/social_determinants/en/.

Yearby, R. (2015). "Sick and Tired of Being Sick and Tired: Putting an End to Separate and Unequal Health Care in the United States 50 Years After the Civil Rights Act of 1964." *Health Matrix: The Journal of Law-Medicine*, 25(1). https://scholarlycommons.law.case.edu/healthmatrix/vol25/iss1/3.

Yun, J., D. Kessler, and D. Glickman. (2019). "We Need Better Answers on Nutrition." *New York Times*, February 28. https://www.nytimes.com/2019/02 /28/opinion/nutrition-health.html.

Zerhouni, Y. A., Q. D. Trinh, S. Lipsitz, J. Goldberg, J. Irani, R. Bleday, A. H. Haider, and N. Melnitchouk. (2019). "Effect of Medicaid Expansion on Colorectal Cancer Screening Rates." *Diseases of the Colon & Rectum*, 62(1), 97-103. doi:10.1097/DCR.0000000000001260.

Chapter 4. How the Game Is Played

Addressing Disparities in Health and Healthcare: Issues of Reform; Hearing Before the Subcommittee on Health of the Committee on Ways and Means US House of Representatives. (2008). 110th Cong. Second session, June 10. http://www.gpo .gov/fdsys/pkg/CHRG-110hhrg47453/pdf/CHRG-110hhrg47453.pdf.

Agency for Healthcare Research and Quality. (2004). *National Healthcare Disparities Report: Summary*. Rockville, MD: Agency for Healthcare Research and Quality. https://archive.ahrq.gov/qual/nhdr03/nhdr03.htm.

——. (2006). *National Healthcare Disparities Report*. Rockville, MD: Agency for Healthcare Research and Quality. https://archive.ahrq.gov/qual/nhdr06 /nhdr06.htm.

——. (2011). *National Healthcare Disparities Report*. Rockville, MD: Agency for Healthcare Research and Quality. https://archive.ahrq.gov/research/findings /nhqrdr/nhdr11/index.html.

——. (2011). *National Healthcare Quality Report*. Rockville, MD: Agency for Healthcare Research and Quality. https://archive.ahrq.gov/research/findings /nhqrdr/nhqr11/index.html.

American Medical Association. (2009). "AMA Supports H.R. 3200, 'America's Affordable Health Choices Act of 2009.'" Press release, July 16. http://www .ama-assn.org/ama/pub/news/news/ama-supports-hr-3200.page.

American Psychological Association. (2009). *Psychological and Behavioral Perspectives on Health Disparities*. Communique, March 2009. Washington,

DC: APA. http://www.apa.org/pi/oema/restheirces/communique/2009/03
/march.pdf.

"Barack Obama's Plan for a Healthy America: Lowering Health Care Costs and
Ensuring Affordable, High-Quality Health Care for All." (n.d.). BarackObama
.com, November 1, 2014. http://www.nytimes.com/packages/pdf/politics
/factsheet_healthcare.pdf.

Baucus, M. (2008). "Finance Chairman Baucus Unveils Blueprint for Comprehensive Health Care Reform." US Senate Committee on Finance. Press release,
November 12. http://www.finance.senate.gov/newsroom/chairman/release
/?id=a36a2265-d3ea-41c3-904c-d02620103acb.

Brandon, K. (2009). "The President on Health Care: 'They Are Going to Get This
Done.'" *White House Blog*, July 17. http://www.whitehouse.gov/blog/The
-President-on-Health-Care-They-are-Going-to-Get-this-Done.

Breakey, W. R., P. J. Fischer, M. Kramer, G. Nestadt, A. J. Romanoski, A. Ross,
R. M. Royall, and O. Stine. (1989). "Health and Mental Health Problems of
Homeless Men and Women in Baltimore." *Journal of the American Medical
Association*, 262, 1352–1357.

Breslau, J., S. Aguilar-Gaxiola, K. S. Kendler, M. Su, D. Williams, and R. C.
Kessler. (2006). "Specifying Race-Ethnic Differences in Risk for Psychiatric
Disorder in a USA National Sample." *Psychological Medicine*, 36(1), 57–68.

Centers for Disease Control and Prevention. (2007). *Health, United States, 2007
with Chartbook on Trends in the Health of Americans*. Hyattsville, MD: CDC,
table 61, 262–263.

———. (2012). *Childhood Obesity Facts*. Hyattsville, MD: CDC. http://www.cdc.gov
/obesity/data/childhood.html.

———. (2012). *Health, United States, 2011: With Special Feature on Socioeconomic
Status and Health*. Hyattsville, MD: National Center for Health Statistics.
http://www.cdc.gov/nchs/data/hus/hus11.pdf#listfigures.

Cochran, S., J. Sullivan, and V. Mays. (2003). "Prevalence of Mental Disorders,
Psychological Distress, and Mental Health Services Use among Lesbian,
Gay, and Bisexual Adults in the United States." *Journal of Consulting and
Clinical Psychology*, 71, 53–61.

Cooper, J., Y. Aratani, J. Knitzer, A. Douglas-Hall, R. Masi, P. Banghart, and S.
Dababnah. (2008). *Unclaimed Children Revisited: The Status of Children's Mental
Health Policy in the United States*. New York: National Center for Children in
Poverty.

Dawes, D. (2013). "Health Reform: A Bridge to Health Equity." In A. M. Culp, ed.,
*Child and Family Advocacy: Bridging the Gaps between Research, Practice, and
Policy*, 35–49. New York: Springer.

Dwyer, J. (2008). "After a Death Seen on Tape, Change Is Promised." *New York
Times*, July 12, 2008. http://www.nytimes.com/2008/07/12/nyregion
/12about.html?_r=0.

Evans, J., and J. Schiff. (2009). "A Timeline of Kennedy's Health Care Achievements and Disappointments." *Kaiser Health News*, August 26. http://www
.kaiserhealthnews.org/stories/2009/august/26/kennedy-health-care-timeline
.aspx.

Executive Order No. 13507. (2009). "Establishment of the White House Office of
Health Reform," April 8. https://www.whitehouse.gov/the-press-office
/executive-order-establishing-white-house-office-health-reform.

"From Camp David, Obama Gets a Public Option Earful." (2009). *Fox News*.
September 4, 2009. https://www.foxnews.com/politics/from-camp-david
-obama-gets-a-public-option-earful.

Garber, K. (2009). "AMA: Healthcare Reform Bill a 'Starting Point.'" *US News*,
July 29, 2009. http://www.usnews.com/news/national/articles/2009/07/29
/ama-healthcare-reform-bill-a-starting-point.

Gergen, D. (2012). "A Candid Conversation with Sandra Day O'Connor: 'I Can
Still Make a Difference.'" *Parade*, September 30. https://parade.com/125604
/davidgergen/30-sandra-day-oconnor-i-can-make-a-difference/.

Institute of Medicine. (2002). *Unequal Treatment: Confronting Racial and Ethnic
Disparities in Healthcare*. Washington, DC: National Academies Press.

———. (2011). *The Health of Lesbian, Gay, Bisexual and Transgender People: Building a
Foundation to Better Health*. Washington, DC: National Academies Press.

———. (2012). *How Far Have They Come in Reducing Health Disparities? Progress
since 2000*. Workshop Summary. Washington, DC: National Academies
Press.

Janssen, I., W. Craig, W. Boyce, and W. Pickett. (2004). "Associations between
Overweight and Obesity with Bullying Behaviors in School-Aged Children."
Pediatrics, 113, 1187–1194.

Kaiser Family Foundation. (2008). "Eliminating Racial/Ethnic Disparities in
Health Care: What Are the Options?" Issue brief, October 2008. https://
www.kff.org/disparities-policy/issue-brief/eliminating-racialethnic
-disparities-in-health-care-what/.

———. (2008). "President Obama's Campaign Position on Health Reform and
Other Health Care Issues." KFF, November 1. http://kff.org/disparities
-policy/issue-brief/president-obamas-campaign-position-on-health-reform/.

Kemper, A. R., G. R. Maslow, S. Hill, B. Namdari, N. M. Allen LaPointe, A. P.
Goode, R. R. Coeytaux, et al. (2018). *Attention Deficit Hyperactivity Disorder:
Diagnosis and Treatment in Children and Adolescents*. Comparative Effectiveness
Review No. 203. Prepared by the Duke University Evidence-Based
Practice Center under Contract No. 290-2015-00004-I. AHRQ Publication
No. 18-EHC005-EF. Rockville, MD: Agency for Healthcare Research and
Quality. https://effectivehealthcare.ahrq.gov/sites/default/files/pdf/cer-203
-adhd-final_0.pdf.

Kennedy, E. (n.d.). *Fighting for Quality, Affordable Health Care*. http://www.tedken nedy.org/service/item/health_care.html.

Kessler, G. (2012). "Sarah Palin, 'Death Panels' and 'Obamacare.'" *Washington Post*, June 27. http://www.washingtonpost.com/blogs/fact-checker/post/sarah -palin-death-panels-and-obamacare/2012/06/27/gJQAysUP7V_blog.html.

Koegel, P. M., A. Burnam, and R. K. Farr. (1988). "The Prevalence of Specific Psychiatric Disorders among Homeless Individuals in the Inner City of Los Angeles." *Archives of General Psychiatry* 45, 1085–1093.

LaVeist, T., D. Gaskin, and P. Richard. (2009). *The Economic Burden of Health Inequalities in the United States*. Washington, DC: Joint Center for Political and Economic Studies.

Lee, J. (2009). "Health Reform: 'Urgency and Determination.'" *White House Blog*, May 3. http://www.whitehouse.gov/blog/Health-Reform-Urgency-and -Determination.

———. (2009). "The President Spells Out His Vision on Health Care Reform." *White House Blog*, June 3. https://www.whitehouse.gov/blog/2009/06/03 /president-spells-out-his-vision-health-care-reform.

Low, N., and J. Hardy. (2007). "Psychiatric Disorder Criteria and Their Applica- tion to Research in Different Racial Groups." *BMC Psychiatry*, 7(1). doi:10.1186/1471-244X-7-1.

Martin, D. (2009). "Obama Calls for Health-Care Reform in 2009." CNN, February 24. http://www.cnn.com/2009/POLITICS/02/24/obama.health .care/index.html?_s=PM:POLITICS.

Minority Health and Health Disparities Research and Education Act of 2000. P.L. 106–525, 114 Stat. 2495.

Murray, S., and P. Kane. (2009). "Pelosi Vows Passage of Health-Care Overhaul." *Washington Post*, July 27. http://www.washingtonpost.com/wp-dyn/content /article/2009/07/26/AR2009072602856.html.

National Alliance on Mental Illness. (2013). "Mental Illness: Facts and Numbers." Arlington, VA. https://namieasysite.com/wp-content/uploads/sites/2/2013 /05/mentalillness_factsheet.pdf.

National Association of State Mental Health Program Directors. (2008). *Measure- ment of Health Status for People with Serious Mental Illnesses*. Alexandria, VA: NASMHPD. http://www.nasmhpd.org/content/measurement-health-status -people-serious-mental-illnesses.

National Federation of Independent Business v. Sebelius, 132 U.S. 2566.

"Nelson for Senate." (2012). *Miami Herald*, October 21.

Newton-Small, J. (2009). "And. Here. They. Go." *Time*, April 20. http://swampland .time.com/2009/04/20/and-here-they-go/.

Obama, B. (2009). "President Obama Calls Health Insurance Reform Key to Stronger Economy and Improvement on Status Quo." Weekly address,

August 8. http://www.whitehouse.gov/the-press-office/theyekly-address
-president-obama-calls-health-insurance-reform-key-stronger-economy-a.

———. (2009). "Remarks by President Obama, HHS Secretary-Designate Kathleen
Sebelius, and White House Office of Health Reform Director Nancy-Ann
DeParle." Press release, March 2. https://www.whitehouse.gov/the-press
-office/remarks-president-obama-hhs-secretary-designate-kathleen-sebelius
-and-white-house-o.

———. (2009). "Remarks by the President at the Opening of the White House
Forum on Health Reform." Press release, March 5. http://www.whitehouse
.gov/the-press-office/remarks-president-opening-white-house-forum-health
-reform.

———. (2009). "Remarks by the President on Senate Passage of Health Insurance
Reform." Press release, December 24. http://www.whitehouse.gov/the-press
-office/remarks-president-senate-passage-health-insurance-reform.

———. (2009). "Remarks by the President to the Annual Conference of the
American Medical Association." Press release, June 15. https://www.white
house.gov/the-press-office/remarks-president-annual-conference-american
-medical-association.

———. (2009). "Text of a Letter from the President to Senator Edward M.
Kennedy and Senator Max Baucus." The White House, June 2. http://www
.whitehouse.gov/the_press_office/Letter-from-President-Obama-to
-Chairmen-Edward-M-Kennedy-and-Max-Baucus.

Obama, B., and J. Biden. (n.d.) "The Obama-Biden Plan." Office of the President-
Elect. http://change.gov/agenda/health_care_agenda/.

Patient Protection and Affordable Care Act. P.L. 111-148.

Pelosi, N. (2010). "Today, They Have the Opportunity to Complete the Great
Unfinished Business of Their Society and Pass Health Insurance Reform for
All Americans." Press release, March 21. http://pelosi.house.gov/news/press
-releases/pelosi-today-they-have-the-opportunity-to-complete-the-great
-unfinished-business.

Roybal-Allard, L. (2009). "Congresswoman Lucille Roybal-Allard, Healthcare
Equality Advocates 'Light the Night' for Reform, Demand Congressional
Action on Disparities." Press release, June 24. http://roybal-allard.house.gov
/news/documentsingle.aspx?DocumentID=134906.

Sack, K., S. Carter, J. Ellis, F. Hossain, and A. McLean. (2012). "Election 2008—
on the Issues: Health Care." New York Times, May 23. http://elections
.nytimes.com/2008/president/issues/health.html.

Schaefer, N. O., and R. Moffit. (2008). The McCain Health Care Plan: More Power to
Families. Washington, DC: The Heritage Foundation. https://www.heritage
.org/health-care-reform/report/the-mccain-health-care-plan-more-power
-families.

Seabrook, A. (2010). "Health Care Overhaul Boosts Pelosi's Clout." NPR, March 29. http://www.npr.org/templates/story/story.php?storyId=125294497.

Seizing the New Opportunity for Health Reform: Hearing of the Committee on Finance. (2008). 110th Congress, 2nd sess., May 6.

"Service Members Home Ownership Tax Act of 2009—Motion to Proceed." (2009). *Congressional Record,* 155(174), S11907-S11967. http://www.gpo.gov /fdsys/pkg/CREC-2009-11-21/html/CREC-2009-11-21-pt1-PgS11907-2.htm.

Smith, E. (2012). "Timeline of the Health Care Law." CNN.com, June 17. http://www.cnn.com/2012/06/17/politics/health-care-timeline/.

Snow, M., and A. Fantz. (2008). "Woman Who Died on Hospital Floor Called 'Beautiful Person.'" CNN, July 3. http://www.cnn.com/2008/US/07/03 /hospital.woman.death/.

Stagman, S., and J. Cooper. (2010). *Children's Mental Health: What Every Policymaker Should Know.* New York: National Center for Children in Poverty.

Substance Abuse and Mental Health Services Administration. (2003). *Risk of Suicide among Hispanic Females Aged 12 to 17.* National Household Survey on Drug Abuse Report. Rockville, MD: Substance Abuse and Mental Health Services Administration. http://www.oas.samhsa.gov/2k3/LatinaSuicide /LatinaSuicide.htm.

Swartz, M., R. Wagner, J. Swanson, B. Burns, L. George, and D. Padgett. (1998). "Administrative Update: Utilization of Services." *Community Mental Health Journal,* 34(2), 133-144.

"Ted Kennedy and Health Care Reform." (2009). *Newsweek,* July 17. https://www .newsweek.com/ted-kennedy-and-health-care-reform-82011.

Teplin, L. A. (1990). "The Prevalence of Severe Mental Disorder among Male Urban Jail Detainees: Comparison with the Epidemiologic Catchment Area Program." *American Journal of Public Health,* 80, 663-669.

Thomas, P. (2009). "White House Summit on Health Care Reform." External memorandum to CCD Health and Long Term Services Task Forces and interested parties, March 10 (in the author's possession).

Thrush, G. (2009). "Black Caucus Pushes Obama on Health Equity." *Politico,* June 8. http://www.politico.com/blogs/glennthrush/0609/Black_Caucus _pushes_Obama_on_health_equity.html.

US Commission on Civil Rights. (2010). *Health Care Disparities: A Briefing before the United States Commission on Civil Rights.* Briefing Report. Washington, DC: Commission on Civil Rights. https://www.usccr.gov/pubs/docs/Healthcare -Disparities.pdf.

US Department of Health and Human Services. (2001). *Mental Health: Culture, Race, and Ethnicity—A Supplement to Mental Health: A Report of the Surgeon General.* Rockville, MD: Department of Health and Human Services.

US Department of Health and Human Services, Advisory Committee on Minority Health, Office of Minority Health. (2009). *Ensuring That Health Care Reform Will Meet the Health Care Needs of Minority Communities and Eliminate Health Disparities: A Statement of Principles and Recommendations.* Rockville, MD: Department of Health and Human Services. http://minorityhealth.hhs .gov/Assets/pdf/Checked/1/ACMH_HealthCareAccessReport.pdf.

US Department of Health and Human Services, New Freedom Commission on Mental Health. (2003). *Achieving the Promise: Transforming Mental Health Care in America—Final Report.* Rockville, MD: Department of Health and Human Services.

US Department of Health and Human Services, Office of Minority Health. (2012). *Native Hawaiian/Other Pacific Islander Profile.* Rockville, MD: Department of Health and Human Services. http://minorityhealth.hhs.gov /templates/content.aspx?lvl=3&lvlID=4&ID=8593.

US Senate Committee on Finance. (2009). "Baucus, Grassley Release Policy Options for Expanding Health Care Coverage." Press release, May 11. http://www.finance.senate.gov/newsroom/chairman/release/?id=e135f9d6 -6140-4d57-87ab-4b80647283ff.

———. (2009). "Finance Leaders Release Health Care Reform Policy Option." Press release, April 28. http://www.finance.senate.gov/newsroom/chairman /release/?id=f8ea4f72-b3af-4c93-8bf1-922f61714dfd.

———. (2009). "Health Care Reform from Conception to Final Passage: Timeline of the Finance Committee's Work to Reform America's Health Care System." http://www.finance.senate.gov/issue/?id=32be19bd-491e-4192-812f-f65215 c1ba65.

Vernez, G. M., M. A. Burnam, E. A. McGlynn, S. Trude, and B. Mittman. (1988). *Review of California's Program for the Homeless Mentally Ill Disabled.* Report No. R3631-CDMH. Santa Monica, CA: RAND.

Wells, K., R. Klap, A. Koike, and C. Sherbourne. (2001). "Ethnic Disparities in Unmet Need for Alcoholism, Drug Abuse, and Mental Health Care." *American Journal of Psychiatry,* 158, 2027-2032.

Wellstone Action. (2005). *Politics the Wellstone Way: How to Elect Progressive Candidates and Win on Issues.* Edited by Bill Lofy. Minneapolis: University of Minnesota Press.

"White House Forum on Health Reform Attendees and Breakout Session Participants." (2009). Press release, March 5. https://www.whitehouse.gov /the-press-office/white-house-forum-health-reform-attendees-and-breakout -session-participants.

Williams, D. R., H. M. González, H. Neighbors, R. Nesse, J. Abelson, J. M. Sweetman, and J. S. Jackson. (2007). "Prevalence and Distribution of Major Depressive Disorder in African Americans, Caribbean Blacks, and Non-

Hispanic Whites: Results from the National Survey of American Life."
Archives of General Psychiatry, 64, 305-315.

Chapter 5. Winning the Game That Never Ends

Agency for Healthcare Research and Quality. (2004). *National Healthcare Dispari-ties Report: Summary*. Rockville, MD: Agency for Healthcare Research and Quality. http://www.ahrq.gov/qual/nhdr03/nhdrsum03.htm.

———. (2006). *National Healthcare Disparities Report*. Rockville, MD: Agency for Healthcare Research and Quality. http://www.ahrq.gov/qual/nhdr06/nhdr06.htm.

———. (2011). *Clinician Summary: Attention Deficit Hyperactivity Disorder in Children and Adolescents*. Rockville, MD: Agency for Healthcare Research and Quality. http://effectivehealthcare.ahrq.gov/ehc/products/191/1149/adhd_clin_fin_to_post.pdf.

———. (2011). *National Healthcare Disparities Report*. Rockville, MD: Agency for Healthcare Research and Quality. http://www.ahrq.gov/qual/qrdr11.htm.

———. (2011). *National Healthcare Quality Report*. Rockville, MD: Agency for Healthcare Research and Quality. http://www.ahrq.gov/qual/qrdr11.htm.

American Psychological Association. (2009). *Psychological and Behavioral Perspectives on Health Disparities*. Communique, March 2009. Washington, DC: APA. http://www.apa.org/pi/oema/resources/communique/2009/03/march.pdf.

Brandon, K. (2009). "The President on Health Care: 'We Are Going to Get This Done.'" *White House Blog*, July 17. http://www.whitehouse.gov/blog/The-President-on-Health-Care-We-are-Going-to-Get-this-Done.

Breakey, W. R., P. J. Fischer, M. Kramer, G. Nestadt, A. J. Romanoski, A. Ross, R. M. Royall, and O. Stine. (1989). "Health and Mental Health Problems of Homeless Men and Women in Baltimore." *Journal of the American Medical Association, 262*, 1352-1357.

Breslau, J., S. Aguilar-Gaxiola, K. Kendler, S. Maxwell, D. Williams, and R. Kessler. (2006). "Specifying Race-Ethnic Differences in Risk for Psychiatric Disorder in a USA National Sample." *Psychological Medicine, 36*(1), 57-68.

Centers for Disease Control and Prevention. (2007). *Health, United States, 2007 with Chartbook on Trends in the Health of Americans*. Hyattsville, MD: CDC, table 61, 262-263.

———. (2012). *Childhood Obesity Facts*. Hyattsville, MD: CDC. http://www.cdc.gov/obesity/data/childhood.html.

———. (2012). *Health, United States, 2011: With Special Feature on Socioeconomic Status and Health*. Hyattsville, MD: National Center for Health Statistics. http://www.cdc.gov/nchs/data/hus/hus11.pdf#listfigures.

Cochran, S., J. Sullivan, and V. Mays. (2003). "Prevalence of Mental Disorders, Psychological Distress, and Mental Health Services Use among Lesbian,

Gay, and Bisexual Adults in the United States." *Journal of Consulting and Clinical Psychology,* 71, 53–61.

Cohn, J. (2010). "How They Did It." *New Republic,* May 21. http://www .newrepublic.com/article/75077/how-they-did-it.

Evans, J., and J. Schiff. (2009). "A Timeline of Kennedy's Health Care Achievements and Disappointments." *Kaiser Health News,* August 26. http://www .kaiserhealthnews.org/stories/2009/august/26/kennedy-health-care-timeline .aspx.

Final Vote Results for Roll Call 165, Patient Protection and Affordable Care Act. http://clerk.house.gov/evs/2010/roll165.xml.

Final Vote Results for Roll Call 887, Affordable Health Care for America Act. http://clerk.house.gov/evs/2009/roll887.xml.

Health Care and Education Reconciliation Act of 2010. P.L. 111–152.

Institute of Medicine. (2009). *Race, Ethnicity, and Language Data: Standardization for Health Care Quality Improvement.* Washington, DC: National Academies Press.

———. (2011). *The Health of Lesbian, Gay, Bisexual and Transgender People: Building a Foundation to Better Health.* Washington, DC: National Academies Press.

———. (2012). *How Far Have We Come in Reducing Health Disparities? Progress since 2000.* Workshop Summary. Washington, DC: National Academies Press.

Janssen, I., W. Craig, W. Boyce, and W. Pickett. (2004). "Associations between Overweight and Obesity with Bullying Behaviors in School-Aged Children." *Pediatrics,* 113(2004), 1187–1194.

Johnson, C. K. (2010). "AARP, AMA Announce Support for Health Care Bill: Largest Doctors and Retiree Groups Backing Legislation." *Huffington Post,* March 19. http://www.huffingtonpost.com/2010/03/19/aarp-ama-announce -support_n_506060.html.

Joint Hearing on Eliminating the Social Security Disability Backlog, Before the Subcommittee on Social Security and Subcommittee on Income Security and Family Support of the House Committee on Ways & Means. (2009). Testimony of Peggy Hathaway, representing the Consortium for Citizens with Disabilities, March 24. http://www.c-c-d.org/fichiers/CCD-W&M-Jt-Subomm-testimony3 -24-09.doc. Story retold by D. Al-Mohamed. (2009). "Why Do We Need Health Reform Anyway?" *Day in Washington: The Disability Policy Podcast,* September. http://dayinwashington.com/?p=350.

Kaiser Family Foundation. (2008). "President Obama's Campaign Position on Health Reform and Other Health Care Issues." KFF, November 1. http://kff .org/disparities-policy/issue-brief/president-obamas-campaign-position-on -health-reform/.

Kennedy, E. (n.d.). *Fighting for Quality, Affordable Health Care.* http://www.ted kennedy.org/service/item/health_care.html.

Koegel, P. M., A. Burnam, and R. K. Farr. (1988). "The Prevalence of Specific Psychiatric Disorders among Homeless Individuals in the Inner City of Los Angeles." *Archives of General Psychiatry*, 45, 1085–1093.

LaVeist, T., D. Gaskin, and P. Richard. (2009). *The Economic Burden of Health Inequalities in the United States*. Washington, DC: Joint Center for Political and Economic Studies.

Lee, J. (2009). "Health Reform: 'Urgency and Determination.'" *White House Blog*, May 3. http://www.whitehouse.gov/blog/Health-Reform-Urgency-and -Determination.

Lovley, E. (2010). "Harry Reid: We'll Wait on Scott Brown for Health Care Vote." *Politico*, January 20. http://www.politico.com/news/stories/0110/31734.html.

Low, N., and J. Hardy. "Psychiatric Disorder Criteria and Their Application to Research in Different Racial Groups." *BMC Psychiatry*, 7(1). doi:10.1186/1471-244X-7-1.

National Alliance on Mental Illness. (2015). "Mental Illness: Facts and Numbers." Arlington, VA, 2013. http://www2.nami.org/factsheets/mentalillness_fact sheet.pdf.

National Association of State Mental Health Program Directors. (2008). *Measurement of Health Status for People with Serious Mental Illnesses*. Alexandria, VA: National Association of State Mental Health Program Directors. http://www.nasmhpd .org/content/measurement-health-status-people-serious-mental-illnesses.

National Federation of Independent Business v. Sebelius, 132 U.S. 2566.

Obama, B. (2009). "Remarks by the President on Senate Passage of Health Insurance Reform." Press release, December 24. http://www.whitehouse.gov /the-press-office/remarks-president-senate-passage-health-insurance-reform.

———. (2009). "Remarks by the President to a Joint Session of Congress on Health Care." Press release, September 9. http://www.whitehouse.gov/the _press_office/Remarks-by-the-President-to-a-Joint-Session-of-Congress-on -Health-Care/.

Obama, B., and J. Biden. (n.d.). "The Obama-Biden Plan." Office of the President-Elect. http://change.gov/agenda/health_care_agenda/.

———. (2009). "Remarks by the President on Senate Passage of Health Insurance Reform." Press release, December 24. http://www.whitehouse.gov/the-press -office/remarks-president-senate-passage-health-insurance-reform.

———. (2010). "Remarks by the President and Vice President on Health Insurance Reform at the Department of the Interior." Press release, March 23. http:// www.whitehouse.gov/the-press-office/remarks-president-and-vice-president -health-insurance-reform-bill-department-interi.

Patient Protection and Affordable Care Act. P.L. 111-148.

Pear, R. (2009). "Senate Passes Health Care Overhaul on Party-Line Vote." *New York Times*, December 24. http://www.nytimes.com/2009/12/25/health /policy/25health.html.

Pear, R., and J. Calmes. (2009). "Obama Aides Aim to Simplify and Scale Back Health Bills." *New York Times*, September 2.

Pelosi, N. (2010). "Today, We Have the Opportunity to Complete the Great Unfinished Business of Our Society and Pass Health Insurance Reform for All Americans." Press release, March 21. http://pelosi.house.gov/news/press-releases/pelosi-today-we-have-the-opportunity-to-complete-the-great-unfinished-business.

Reid, H. (2009). "Historic Health Reform Vote Marks a New Beginning to Deal with Old Challenges." US Senate Democrats. Press release, December 24. http://democrats.senate.gov/2009/12/24/reid-historic-health-reform-vote-marks-a-new-beginning-to-deal-with-old-challenges/#.U9qOhrHGujo.

Sack, K., S. Carter, J. Ellis, F. Hossain, and A. McLean. (2012). "Election 2008—on the Issues: Health Care." *New York Times*, May 23. http://elections.nytimes.com/2008/president/issues/health.html.

Saslow, E., and P. Rucker. (2010). "Ted Kennedy Is Celebrated for His Longtime Support of Health-Care Reform." *Washington Post*, March 24. http://www.washingtonpost.com/wp-dyn/content/article/2010/03/23/AR2010032303883.html.

"Service Members Home Ownership Tax Act of 2009—Motion to Proceed." (2009). *Congressional Record*, 155(174), S11907–S11967. http://www.gpo.gov/fdsys/pkg/CREC-2009-11-21/html/CREC-2009-11-21-pt1-PgS11907-2.htm.

Shaw, D. (2009). "Senate Passes Historic Bill to Reform the U.S. Health Care System." *OpenCongress* (blog), December 24. http://www.opencongress.org/articles/view/1421-Senate-Passes-Historic-Bill-to-Reform-the-U-S-Health-Care-System.

Stagman, S., and J. Cooper. (2010). *Children's Mental Health: What Every Policymaker Should Know*. New York: National Center for Children in Poverty.

Stewart, M. (2009). "Bachmann: House Dems 'Embarrassed' by Their Health Care Bill." CNN, October 6. http://politicalticker.blogs.cnn.com/2009/10/06/bachmann-house-dems-embarrassed-by-their-health-care-bill/comment-page-7/.

Substance Abuse and Mental Health Services Administration. (2003). *Risk of Suicide among Hispanic Females Aged 12 to 17*. National Household Survey on Drug Abuse Report. Rockville, MD: Substance Abuse and Mental Health Services Administration. http://www.oas.samhsa.gov/2k3/LatinaSuicide/LatinaSuicide.htm.

Swartz, M., R. Wagner, J. Swanson, B. Burns, L. George, and D. Padgett. (1998). "Administrative Update: Utilization of Services." *Community Mental Health Journal*, 34(2), 133–144.

Teplin, L. A. (1990). "The Prevalence of Severe Mental Disorder among Male Urban Jail Detainees: Comparison with the Epidemiologic Catchment Area Program." *American Journal of Public Health*, 80, 663–669.

Thomas, P. (2009). "White House Summit on Health Care Reform." External memorandum to CCD Health and Long Term Services Task Forces and interested parties, March 10 (in the author's possession).

Thrush, G. (2009). "Black Caucus Pushes Obama on Health Equity." *Politico*, June 8. http://www.politico.com/blogs/glennthrush/0609/Black_Caucus _pushes_Obama_on_health_equity.html.

US Commission on Civil Rights. (1999). *The Health Care Challenge: Acknowledging Disparity, Confronting Discrimination, and Ensuring Equality.* Vol. 1: *The Role of Governmental and Private Health Care Programs.* Washington, DC: Commission on Civil Rights.

US Department of Health and Human Services. (2001). *Mental Health: Culture, Race, and Ethnicity—A Supplement to Mental Health: A Report of the Surgeon General.* Rockville, MD: Department of Health and Human Services.

———. (2011). *HHS Action Plan to Reduce Racial and Ethnic Health Disparities: A Nation Free of Disparities in Health and Health Care.* Rockville, MD: Department of Health and Human Services.

US Department of Health and Human Services, Advisory Committee on Minority Health, Office of Minority Health. (2009). *Ensuring That Health Care Reform Will Meet the Health Care Needs of Minority Communities and Eliminate Health Disparities: A Statement of Principles and Recommendations.* Rockville, MD: Department of Health and Human Services. http://minority health.hhs.gov/Assets/pdf/Checked/1/ACMH_HealthCareAccessReport .pdf.

US Department of Health and Human Services, New Freedom Commission on Mental Health. (2003). *Achieving the Promise: Transforming Mental Health Care in America—Final Report.* Rockville, MD: Department of Health and Human Services.

US Department of Health and Human Services, Office of Minority Health. (2012). *Native Hawaiian /Other Pacific Islander Profile.* Rockville, MD: Department of Health and Human Services. http://minorityhealth.hhs.gov /templates/content.aspx?lvl=3&lvlID=4&ID=8593.

US Senate Committee on Finance. (2009). "Baucus Opening Statement at Mark-Up of the America's Healthy Future Act." Press release, October 13. http://www.finance.senate.gov/newsroom/chairman/release/?id=a2728d6d -ecf6-45fa-903f-d2a430147156.

———. (n.d.). "Health Care Reform from Conception to Final Passage: Timeline of the Finance Committee's Work to Reform America's Health Care System." http://www.finance.senate.gov/issue/?id=32be19bd-491e-4192-812f -f65215c1ba65.

US Senate Roll Call Votes. 111th Congress, first Session. H.R. 359. http://www .senate.gov/legislative/LIS/roll_call_lists/roll_call_vote_cfm.cfm?congress =111&session=1&vote=00396.

Vernez, G. M., M. A. Burnam, E. A. McGlynn, S. Trude, and B. Mittman. (1988). *Review of California's Program for the Homeless Mentally Ill Disabled.* Report No. R3631-CDMH. Santa Monica, CA: RAND.

Waidmann, T. (2009). *Estimating the Cost of Racial and Ethnic Health Disparities.* Washington, DC: Urban Institute.

Weir, B. (2009). "Nancy Pelosi Fights for Health Care Reform." *ABC News,* October 31. http://abcnews.go.com/GMA/Weekend/nancy-pelosi-works -hard-health-care-reform/story?id=8961771&page=2.

Wells, K., R. Klap, A. Koike, and C. Sherbourne. (2001). "Ethnic Disparities in Unmet Need for Alcoholism, Drug Abuse, and Mental Health Care." *American Journal of Psychiatry,* 158, 2027–2032.

"White House Forum on Health Reform Attendees and Breakout Session Participants." (2009). Press release, March 5. https://www.whitehouse.gov /the-press-office/white-house-forum-health-reform-attendees-and-breakout -session-participants.

Williams, D., H. Gonzalez, H. Neighbors, R. Nesse, J. Abelson, J. Sweetman, and J. Jackson. (2007). "Prevalence and Distribution of Major Depressive Disorder in African Americans, Caribbean Blacks, and Non-Hispanic Whites: Results from the National Survey of American Life." *Archives of General Psychiatry,* 64, 305–315.

Winerman, L. "House Votes Cap Day of Debate on Health Reform." (2010). *NewsHour,* March 21. http://www.pbs.org/newshour/rundown/as-floor -debate-begins-democrats-predict-health-reform-will-pass/.

Chapter 6. Growing Pains

Congressional Budget Office. (2017). "American Healthcare Act Cost Estimate," March 13. https://www.cbo.gov/sites/default/files/115th-congress-2017-2018 /costestimate/americanhealthcareact.pdf.

Kliff, S. (2017). "Obamacare Is Getting More Popular by the Day." *Vox,* April 25. https://www.vox.com/policy-and-politics/2017/4/25/15419512/obamacare -poll-popular.

Plott, E. (2017). "Eric Cantor: 'If You've Got That Anger Working for You, You're Gonna Let It Be.'" *Washingtonian,* July 26. https://www.washingtonian.com /2017/07/26/eric-cantor-republicans-obamacare-donald-trump/.

Rogin, A. (2016). "States Won by Trump Have Highest 'Obamacare' Enrollment." *ABCNews.com,* December 22.

Taylor, J. (2017). "Trump, McConnell Point Fingers over Health Care Failure." NPR, August 9. http://www.npr.org/2017/08/09/542464074/trump-mcconnell -point-fingers-over-health-care-failure.

Chapter 7. The Future of Health Equity Begins and Ends with the Political Determinants of Health

Centers for Disease Control and Prevention. (2018). "Legionnaires' Disease Signs and Symptoms." https://www.cdc.gov/legionella/about/signs-symptoms .html.

CNN Library. (2019). "Flint Water Crisis Fast Facts." CNN, July 2. https://www .cnn.com/2016/03/04/us/flint-water-crisis-fast-facts/index.html.

Fonger, R. (2017). "Former Flint EM: 'My Job Did Not Include Ensuring Safe Drinking Water.'" MLive, May 2. https://www.mlive.com/news/flint/2017/05 /former_flint_em_my_job_did_not.html.

Goodin-Smith, O. (2018). "Flint's History of Emergency Management and How It Got to Financial Freedom." MLive, https://www.mlive.com/news/flint/2018 /01/city_of_the_state_flints_histo.html.

Harris, A. (2018). "Climate Gentrification: Is Sea Rise Turning Miami High Ground into a Hot Commodity?" Miami Herald. https://www.miamiherald .com/news/local/environment/article222547640.html.

Harvard T.H. Chan School of Public Health, Robert Wood Johnson Foundation, and National Public Radio. (2018). "Discrimination in America: Final Summary." Harvard Opinion Research Program, Cambridge, MA. https:// cdn1.sph.harvard.edu/wp-content/uploads/sites/94/2018/01/NPR-RWJF -HSPH-Discrimination-Final-Summary.pdf.

Hersher, R., and R. Benincasa. (2019). "How Federal Disaster Money Favors the Rich." All Things Considered, March 5. https://www.npr.org/2019/03/05 /688786177/how-federal-disaster-money-favors-the-rich?utm_source=npr _newsletter.

Institute of Medicine. (1981). Health Care in a Context of Civil Rights. Washington, DC: National Academies Press. https://doi.org/10.17226/18680.

Jones, D. K. (2019). "Political Participation in the Least Healthy Place in America: Examining the Political Determinants of Health in the Mississippi Delta." Journal of Health Politics, Policy & Law, 44(3), 505–531. doi:10.1215/03616878-7367048.

King, M. L. (1963). "MLK at Western." Dr. Martin Luther King Jr. [December 18,] 1963 Speech Found. Western Michigan University Archives and Regional History Collections and University Libraries. https://wmich.edu/sites /default/files/attachments/MLK.pdf.

Klein, C., and S. Zellmer. (2016). "Unnatural Disasters and Environmental Injustice." OUPblog. Oxford University Press, April 6. https://blog.oup.com /2016/04/flint-water-crisis-racial-inequality/.

Marmot, M. (2019). "Health Equity in England: The Marmot Review 10 Years On." Interview by Jennifer Dixon of The Health Foundation in London. YouTube, February 26. https://www.youtube.com/watch?v=vp9wPDrMDRU.

Matthew, D. (2015). *Just Medicine: A Cure for Racial Inequality in American Health Care*. New York: New York University Press.

McClelland, E. (2018). "Dayne Walling Flipped the Switch That Set Off the Flint Water Crisis: Now, He's Trying to Make a Comeback." Letter from Michigan. *Politico Magazine*, August 5. https://www.politico.com/magazine/story/2018/08/05/flint-water-crisis-dayne-walling-mayor-state-representative-2018-219078.

McGraw, G. (2018). "For Millions of Americans, Lack of Access to Water Isn't Just a Drought Problem." *Los Angeles Times*. https://www.latimes.com/opinion/op-ed/la-oe-mcgraw-water-poverty-data-20180322-story.html#%E2%80%9D.

McKay, B. (2019). "Heart Attack at 49—America's Biggest Killer Makes a Deadly Comeback." *Wall Street Journal*, June 21.

Michigan Civil Rights Commission. (2017). *The Flint Water Crisis: Systemic Racism through the Lens of Flint*. February 17. Detroit: Michigan Department of Civil Rights. https://www.michigan.gov/documents/mdcr/VFlintCrisisRep-F-Edited3-13-17_554317_7.pdf.

Oppenheimer, G. M., and I. D. Benrubi. (2014). "McGovern's Senate Select Committee on Nutrition and Human Needs versus the Meat Industry on the Diet-Heart Question (1976–1977)." *American Journal of Public Health*, 104(1), 59–69. doi:10.2105/AJPH.2013.301464.

"Our History." (n.d.). Healthy Flint Research Coordinating Center. https://www.hfrcc.org/about/.

Peretti, J. (2012). "Why Our Food Is Making Us Fat." *The Guardian*, June 11.

Satcher, D., G. E. Fryer, J. McCann, A. Troutman, S. H. Woolf, and G. Rust. (2005). "What If We Were Equal? A Comparison of the Black-White Mortality Gap in 1960 and 2000." *Health Affairs*, 24(2), 459–464. https://doi.org/10.1377/hlthaff.24.2.459.

Senterfitt, J. W., A. Long, M. Shih, and S. M. Teutsch. (2013). *How Social and Economic Factors Affect Health*. Social Determinants of Health No. 1. Los Angeles: Los Angeles County Department of Public Health. http://publichealth.lacounty.gov/epi/docs/SocialD_Final_Web.pdf.

Solly, M. (2018). "United States Drops 21 Spots in Global Life Expectancy Rankings." Smithsonian.com, October 19. https://www.smithsonianmag.com/smart-news/united-states-drops-21-places-global-life-expectancy-rankings-180970585/.

Wang, Y. C., K. McPherson, T. Marsh, S. L. Gortmaker, and M. Brown. (2011). "Health and Economic Burden of the Projected Obesity Trends in the USA and the UK." *The Lancet*, 378, 815–825.

Wellstone, P. (2012). "Paul Welstone Quotes." https://www.wellstone.org/legacy/speeches/paul-wellstone-quotes.

White, A., and D. Chanoff. (2011). *Seeing Patients: Unconscious Bias in Health Care.* Cambridge, MA: Harvard University Press.

Whiteman, H. (2014). "Worldwide Obesity Rates See 'Startling' Increase over Past 3 Decades." *Medical News Today,* May 29. https://www .medicalnewstoday.com/articles/277450.php.

Woolf, S. H., R. E. Johnson, G. E. Fryer Jr., G. Rust, and D. Satcher. (2004). "The Health Impact of Resolving Racial Disparities: An Analysis of U.S. Mortality Data." *American Journal of Public Health,* 94(12), 2078-2081.

Index

About the Author

Daniel E. Dawes, an attorney, professor, and author, is the director of the Satcher Health Leadership Institute at Morehouse School of Medicine in Atlanta, Georgia, and cofounder of the Health Equity Leadership and Exchange Network (HELEN). Dawes's research focuses on health inequities among under-resourced, vulnerable, and marginalized communities. He brings a forward-thinking, inclusive, and multidisciplinary approach to the law and public policy and has been at the forefront of recent major federal health policy negotiations in the United States.

Among his many achievements, he was an instrumental figure in shaping the Mental Health Parity Act, the Genetic Information Nondiscrimination Act, the Americans with Disabilities Act Amendments Act, and the Affordable Care Act ("ObamaCare"). A published expert on health reform, health equity, health disparities, mental/behavioral health, and the social determinants of health, Dawes is the author of the groundbreaking book, *150 Years of ObamaCare*, published by Johns Hopkins University Press, which has received critical acclaim and endorsements from a bipartisan group of national leaders.

An elected fellow of the New York Academy of Medicine, Dawes serves on several boards, commissions, and councils focused on improving health outcomes and elevating health equity in the United States and around the world, including the Centers for Disease Control and Prevention (CDC) Federal Advisory Committee on Health Disparities, Robert Wood Johnson Foundation's Policies for Action National Advisory Committee, the Hogg Foundation for Mental Health National Advisory Council, the Healthcare Georgia Foundation Board of Directors, the Alliance for Strong Families and Communities Board of Directors, the New York City Department of Health & Mental Hygiene Mental Health Advisory Group, and the Children's Mental Health Network National Advisory Council.

He is the recipient of several national awards and recognition, including the American Public Health Association's Medical Care Section Award for Significant Contribution to Public Health, the Centers for Disease Control and Prevention's Health Equity Champion Award, the American Psychological Association's Exceptional Leadership in Advocacy Award, Families USA Health Equity Advocate Award, the National Medical Association's Louis Stokes Health Policy Award, Gift of Life Healthcare Vanguard Award, and the SHIRE Health Reform Champion Award. Dawes received his juris doctor degree from the University of Nebraska.

Website: www.DanielEDawes.com
Twitter: @DanielEDawes
LinkedIn: www.linkedin.com/in/danieldawes/